Let's Get HEALTHY!

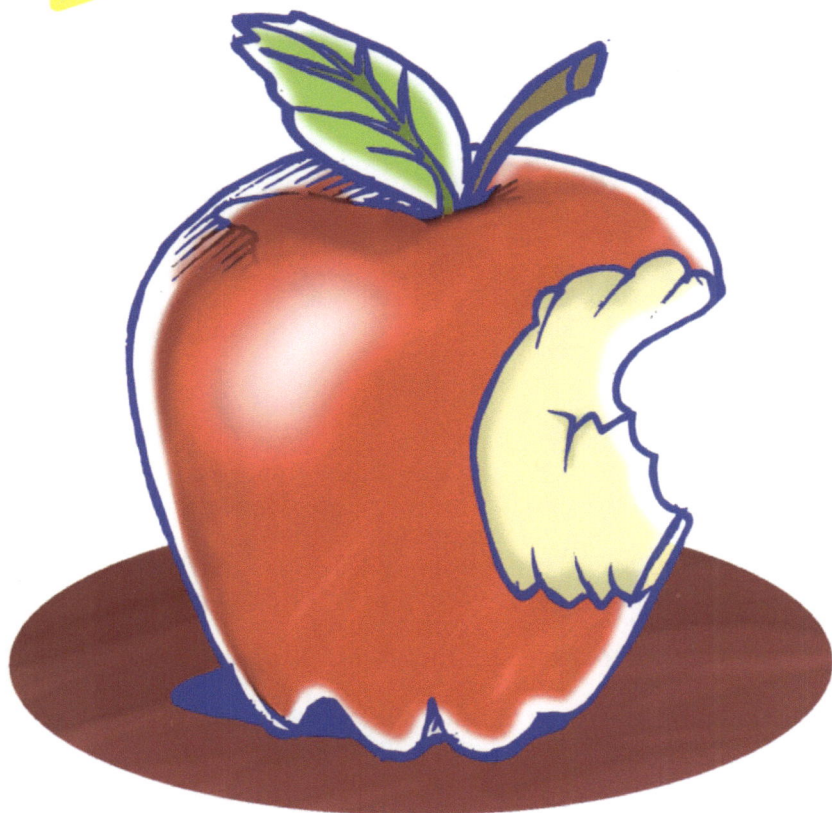

I0116371

Kimberly Sandefur

Illustration by Coz Evan
Edited by Daniel Alfaro

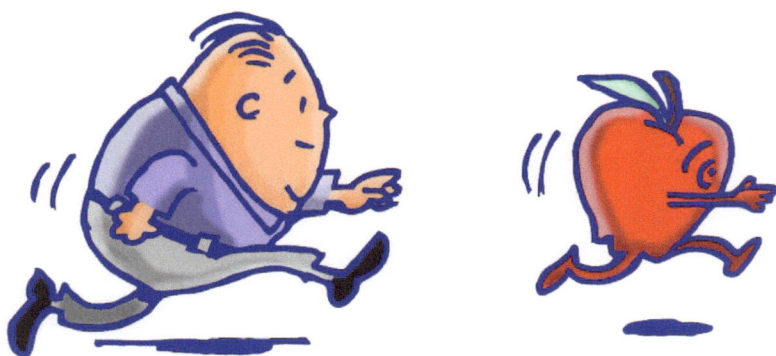

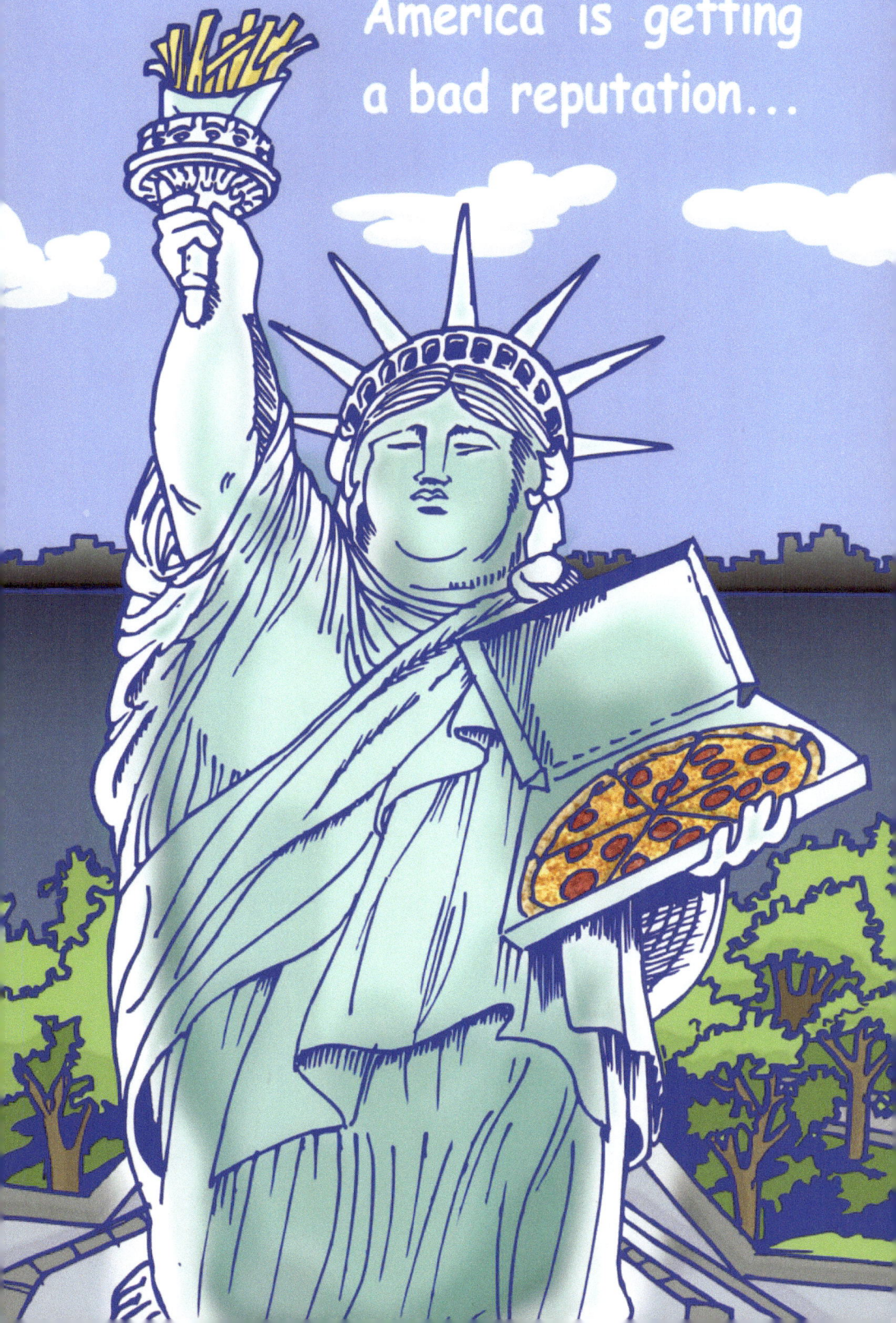

America is getting
a bad reputation...

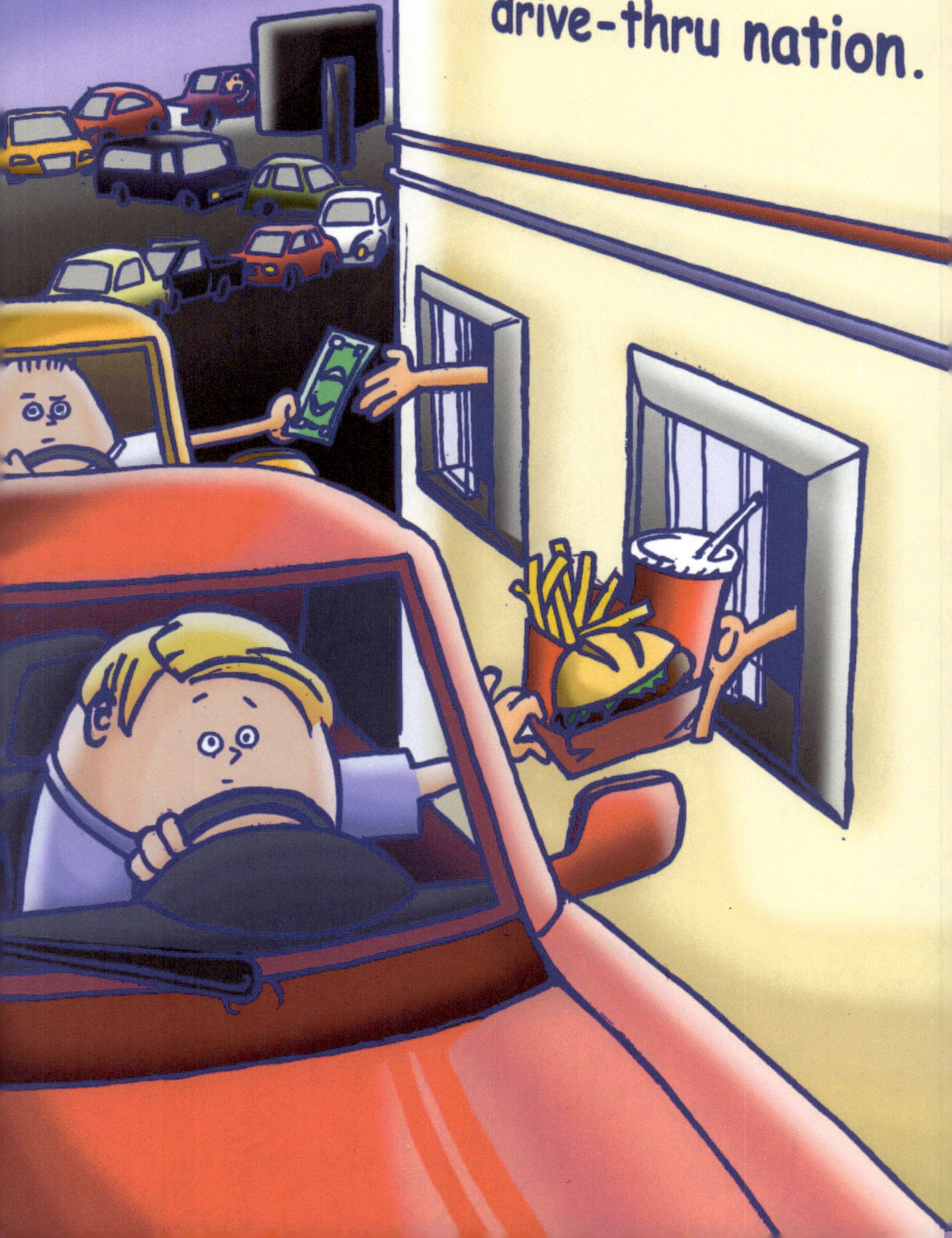

of being a supersized, drive-thru nation.

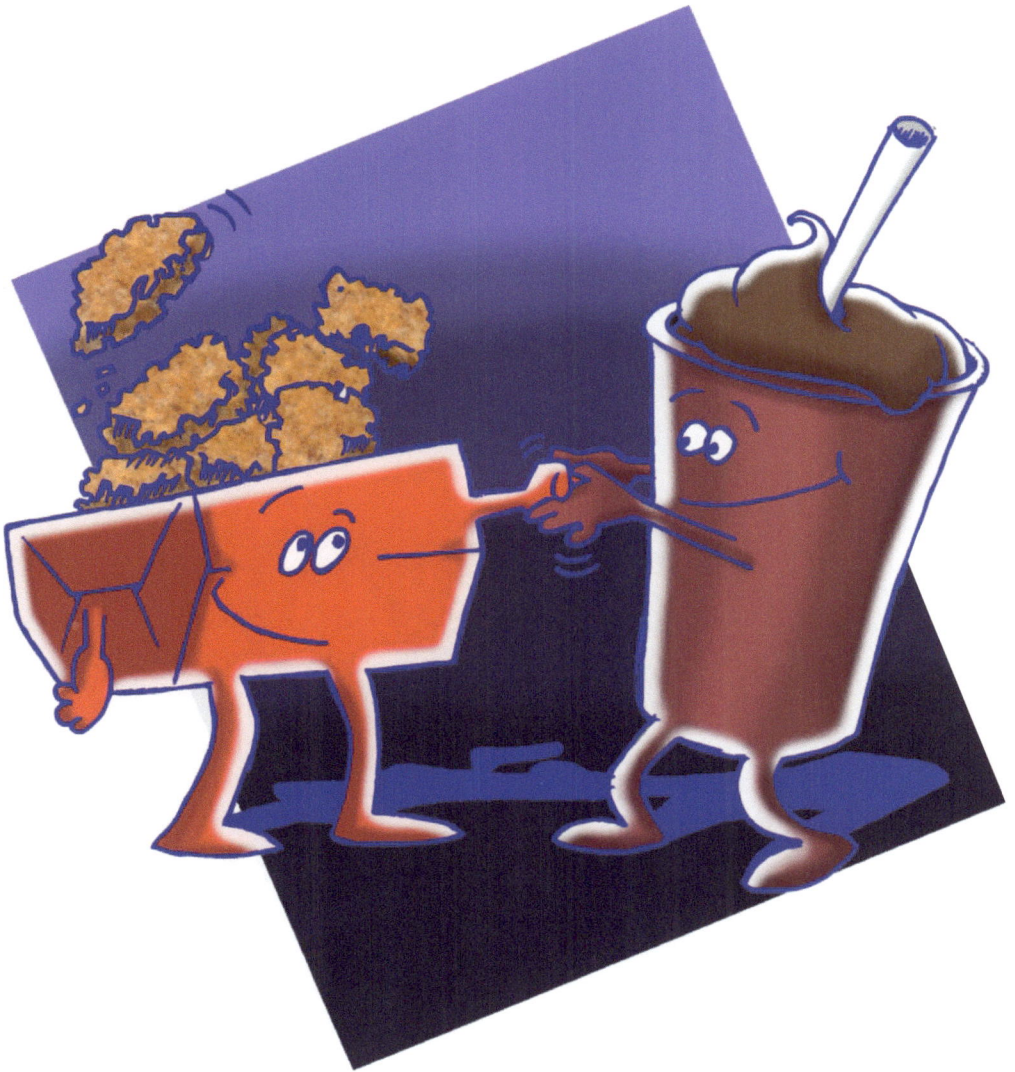

We live off of burgers,
chicken nuggets and shakes.

We're killing ourselves
with every bite that we take!

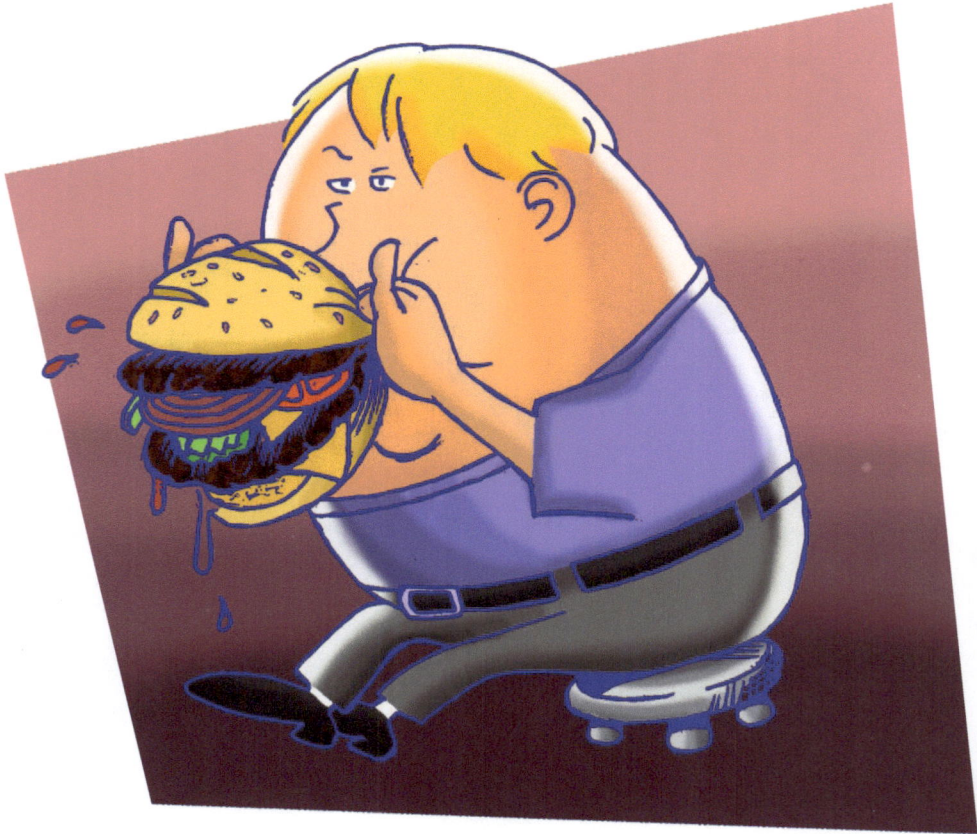

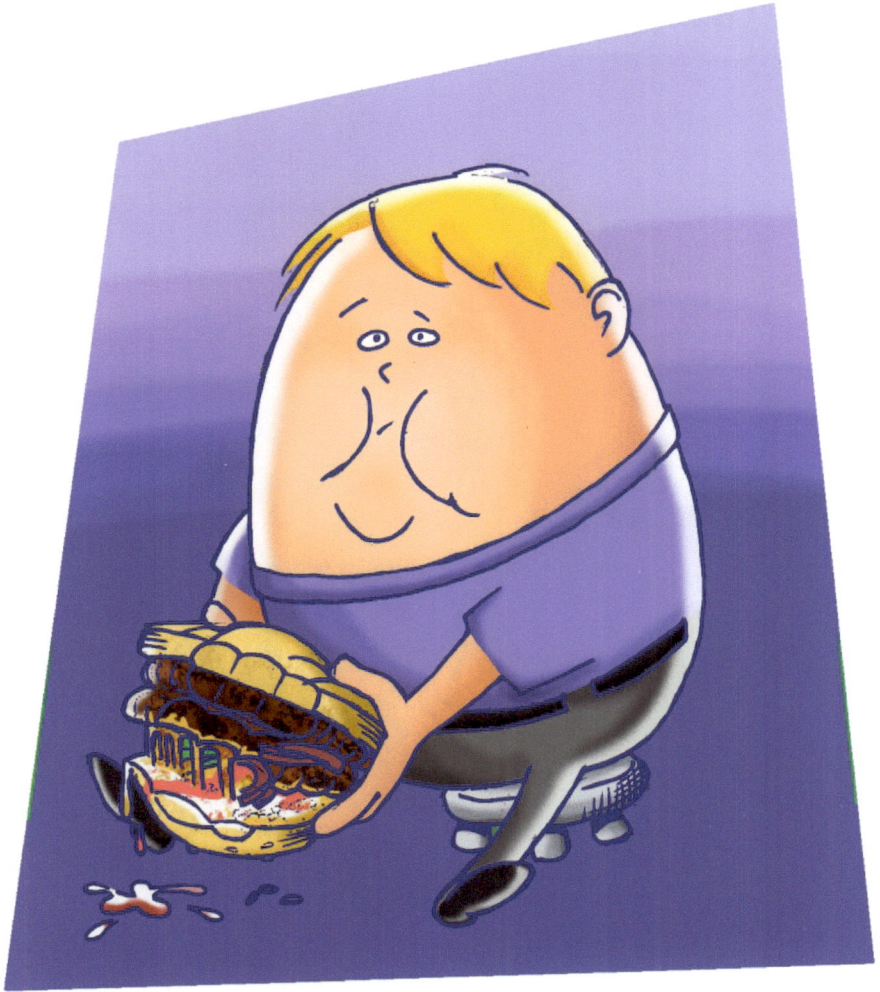

Well sit down and
listen to what I have to say.

We need to start making life changes today!

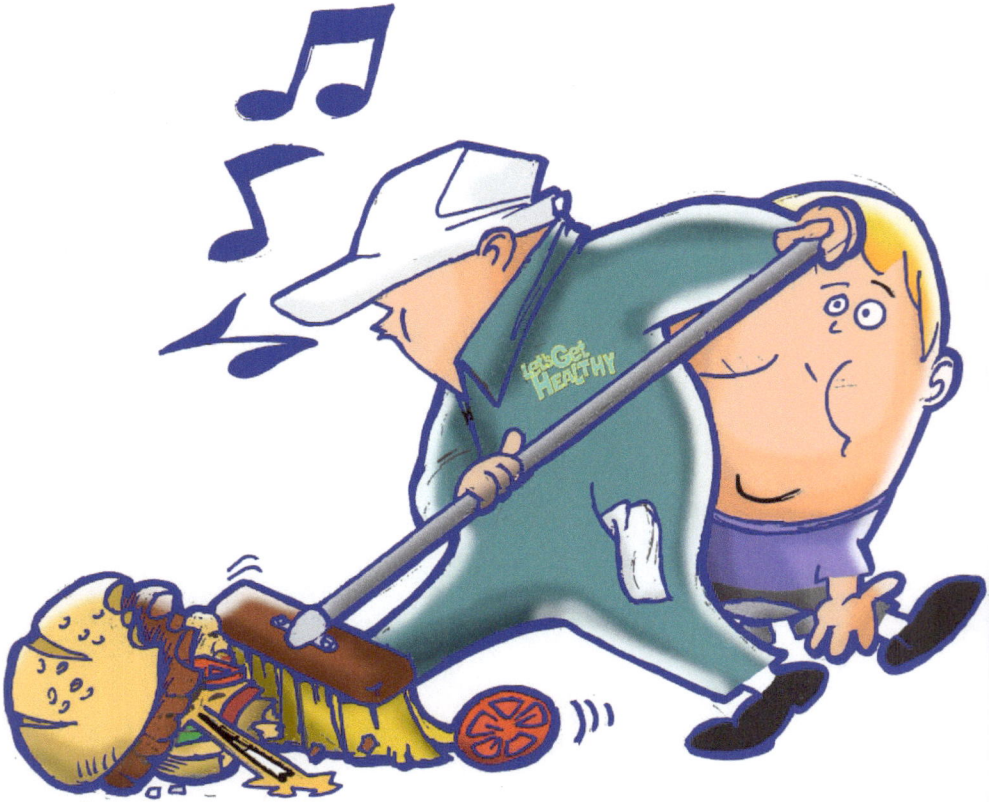

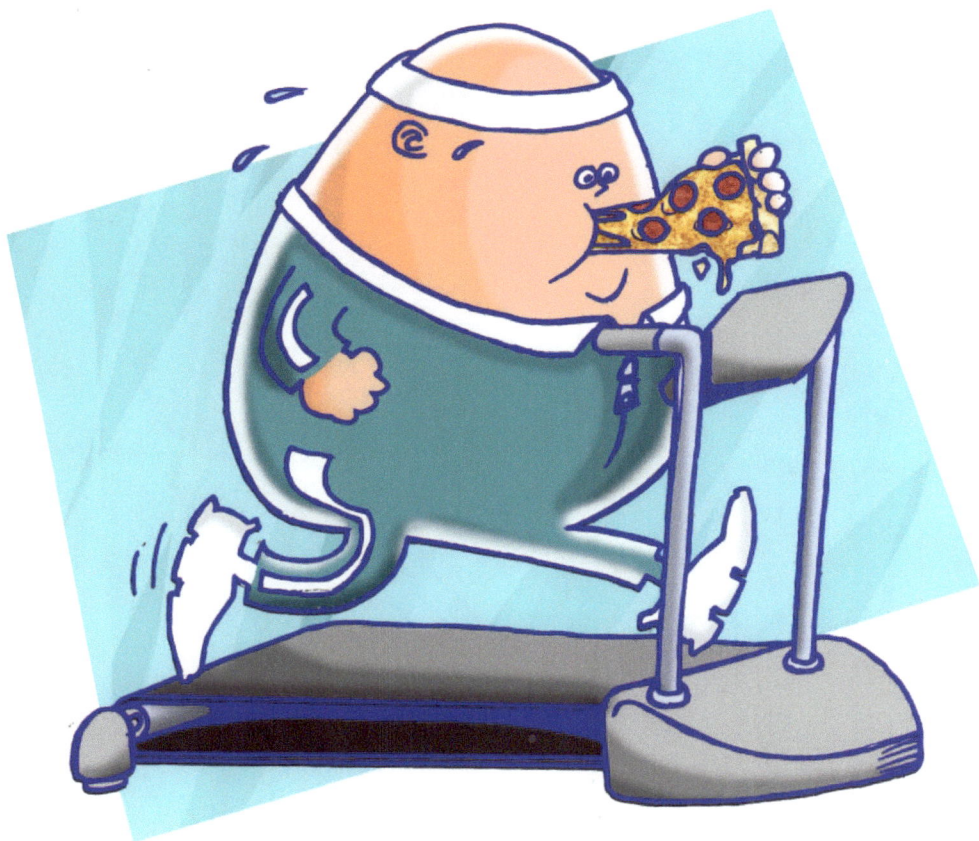

We want to lose
weight and want to be thin...

But pizza and cheesecake

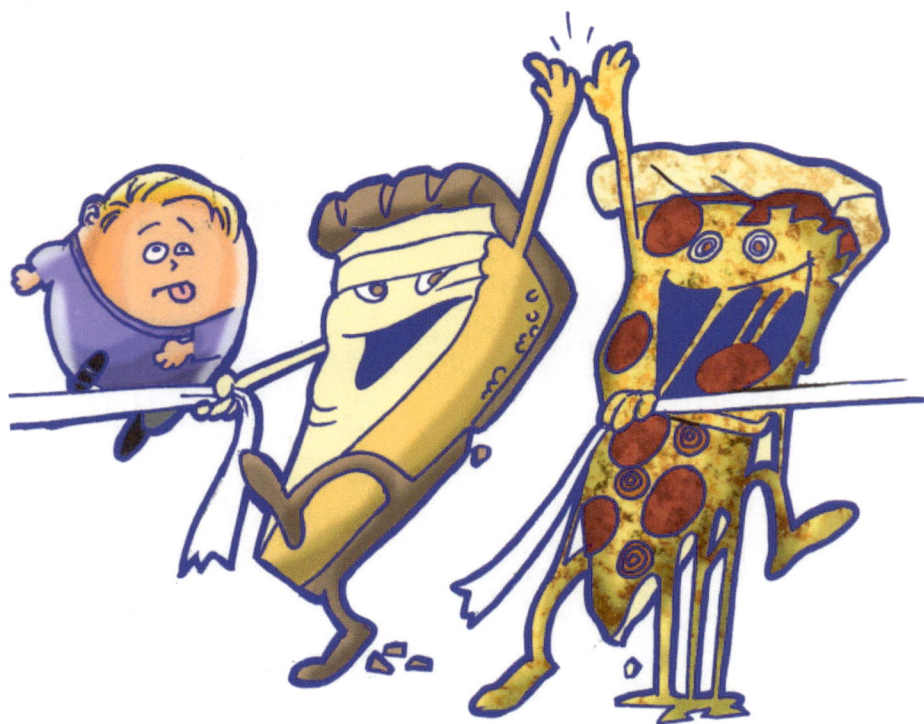

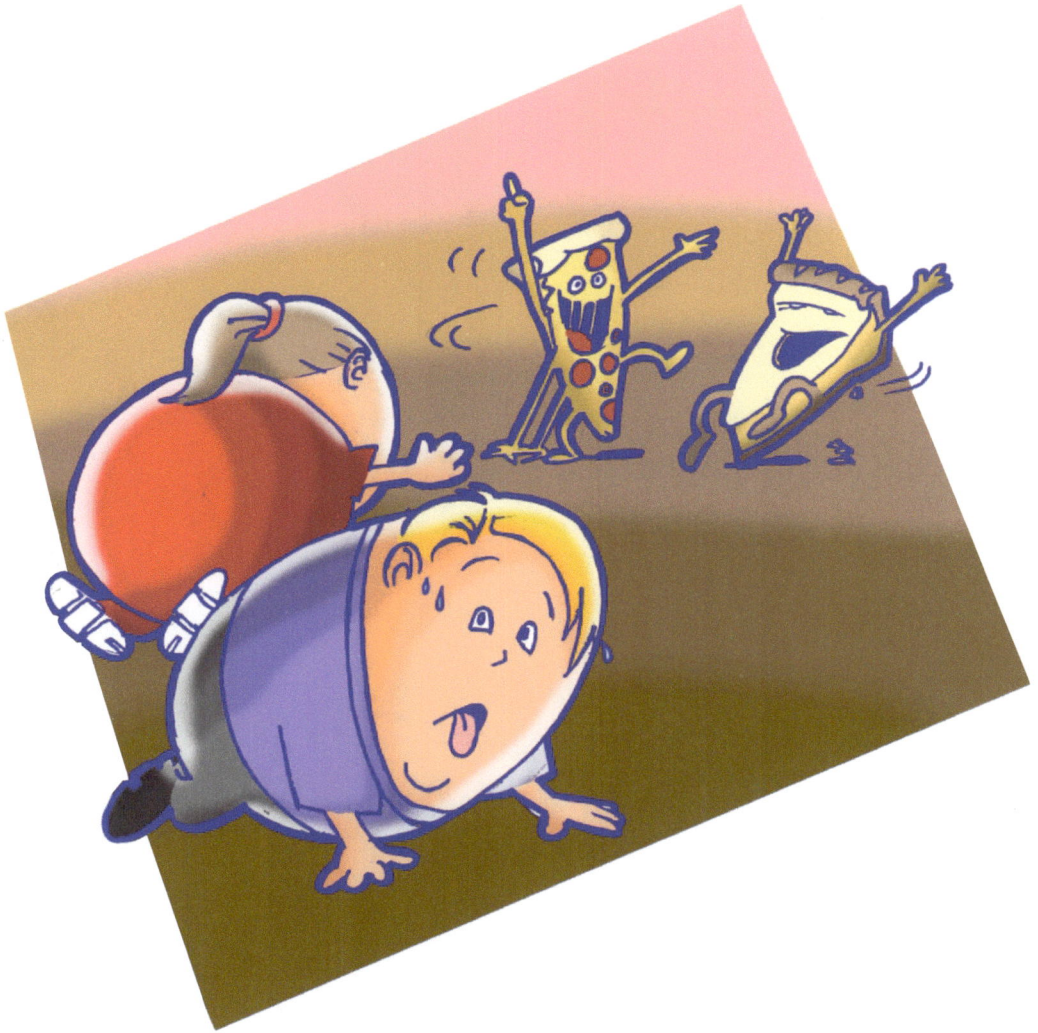

...won't help us win!

Our butts are
so big and our
bellies are round,

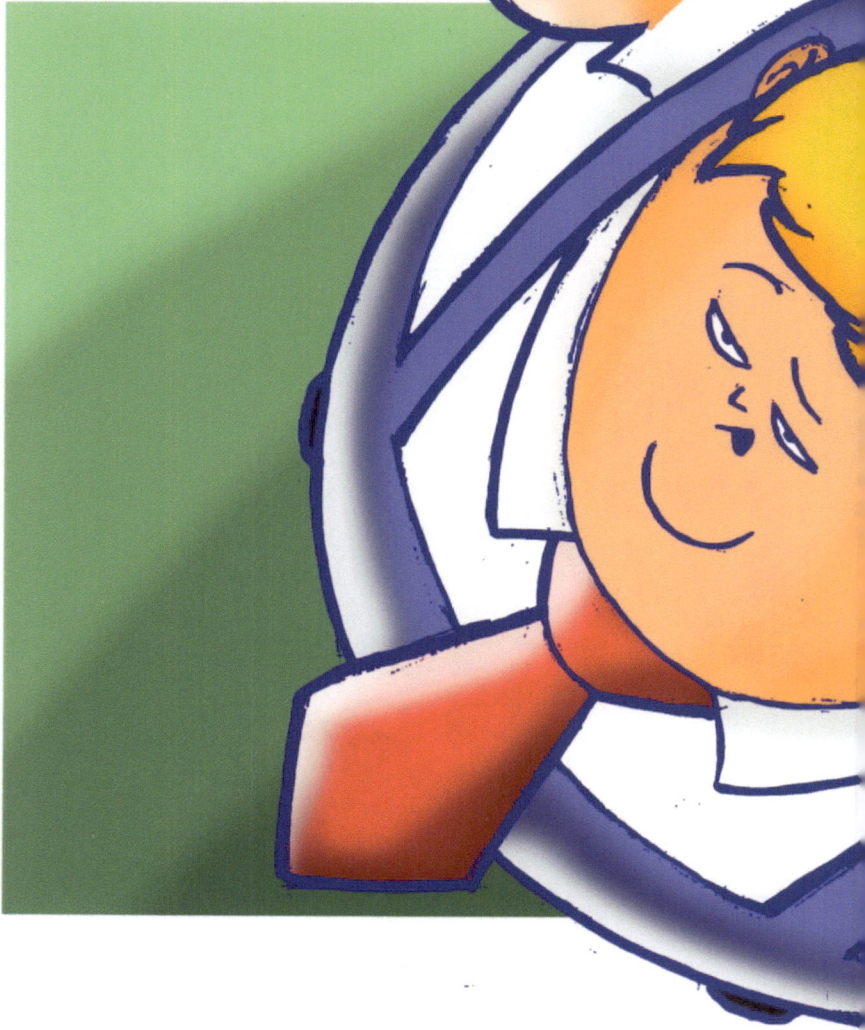

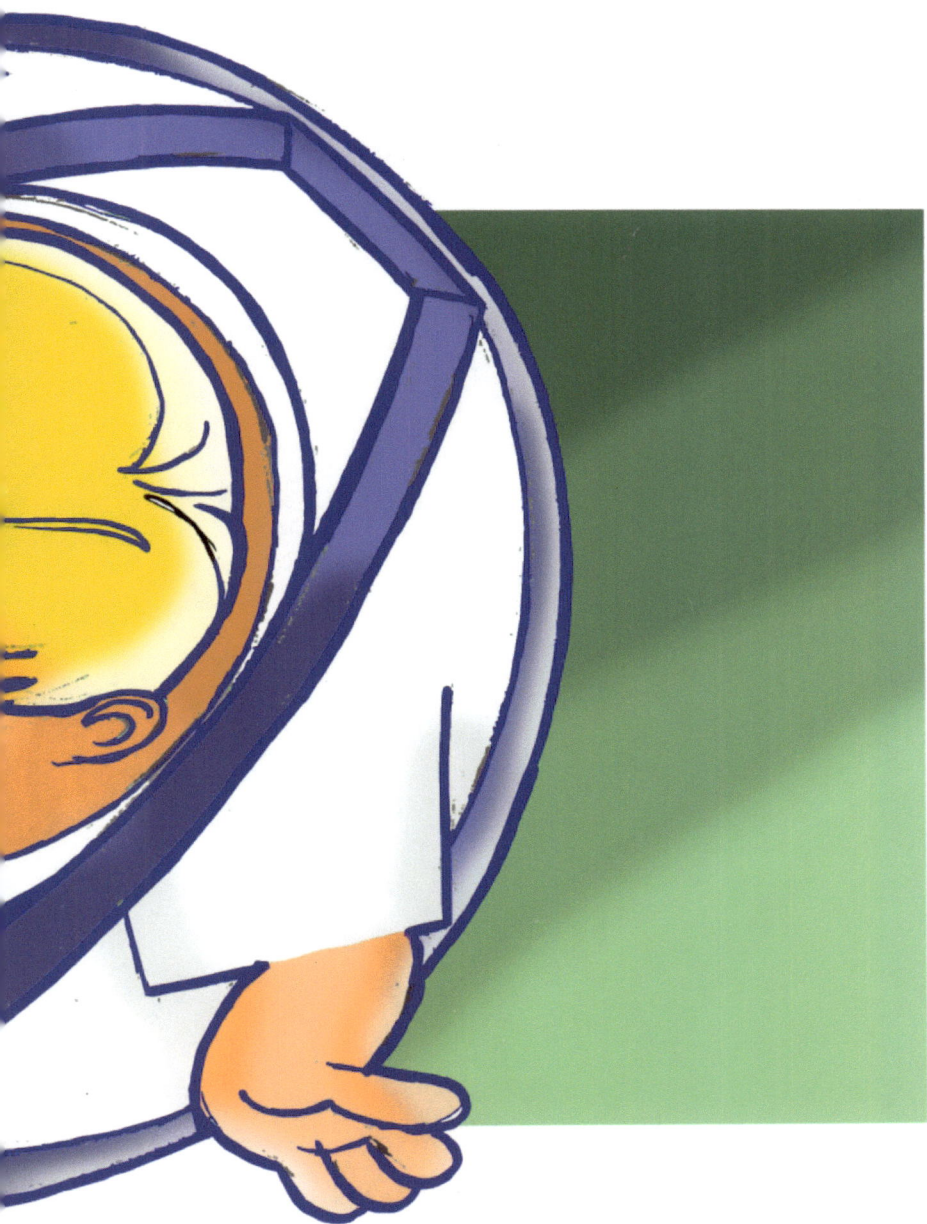

we can't even see
our feet on the ground!

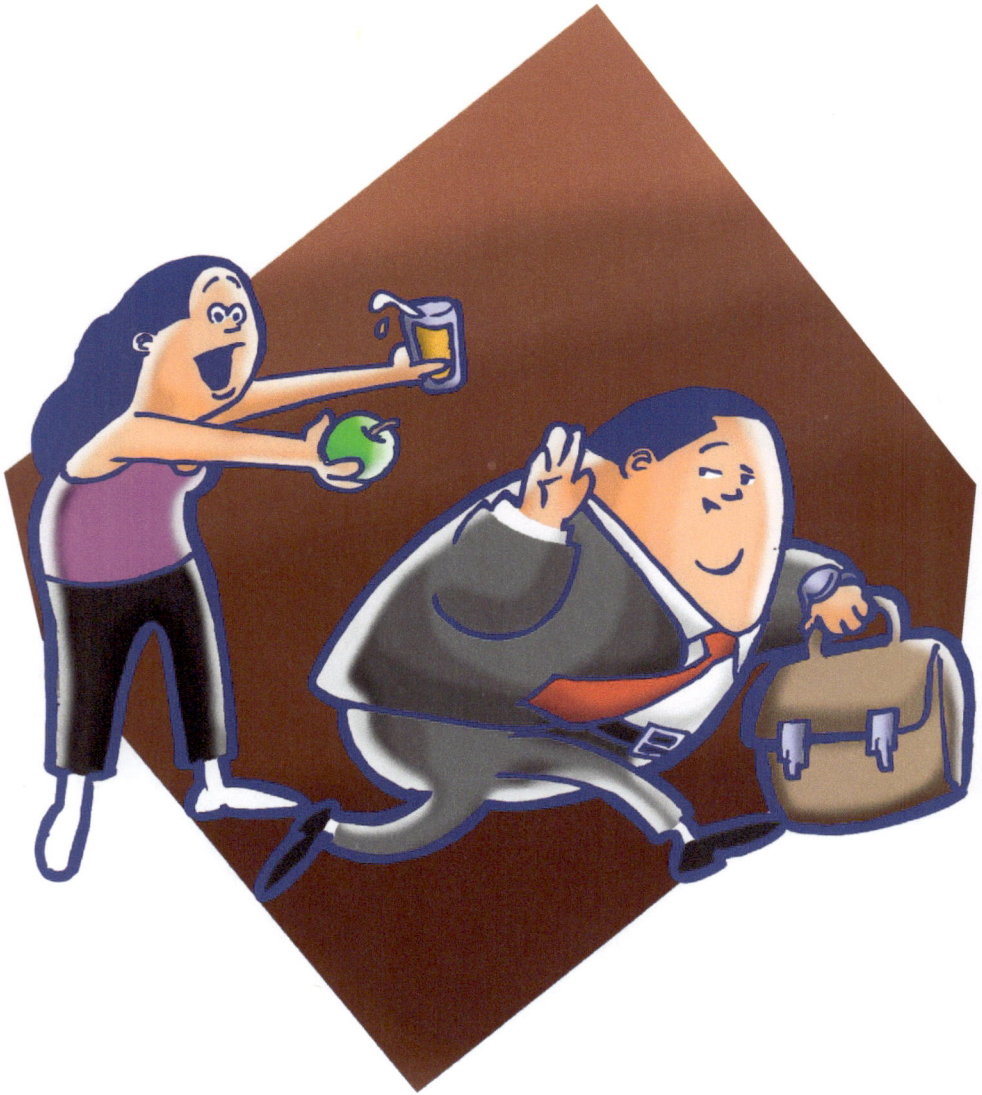

We fast all through
morning and won't eat a bite.

By lunch we are starving so we eat until night.

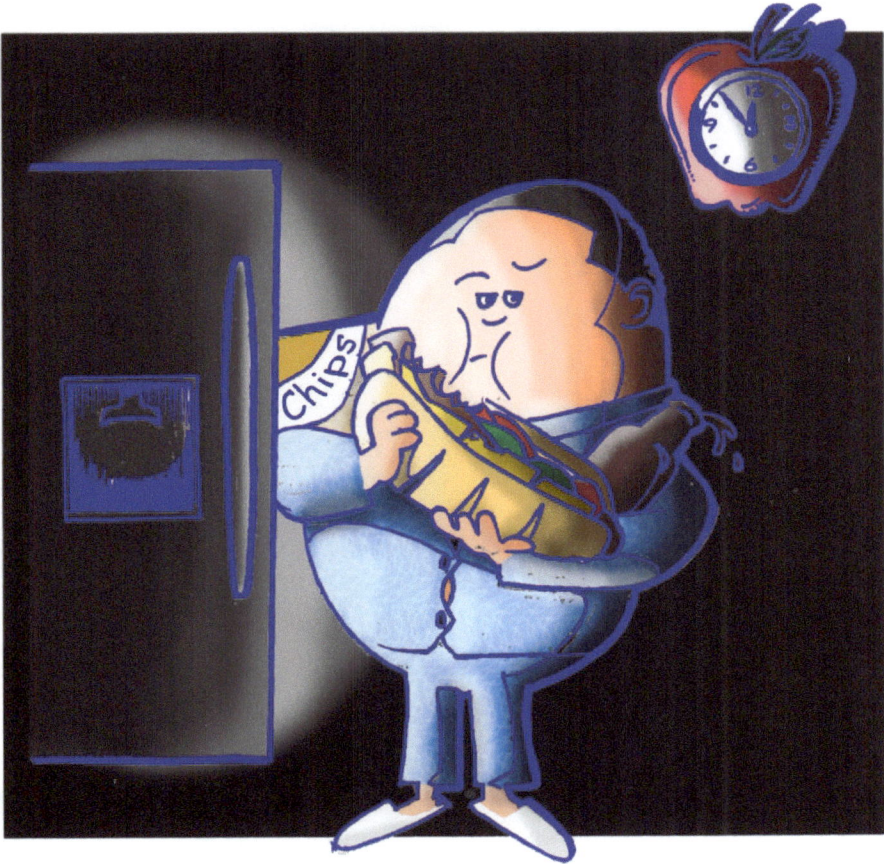

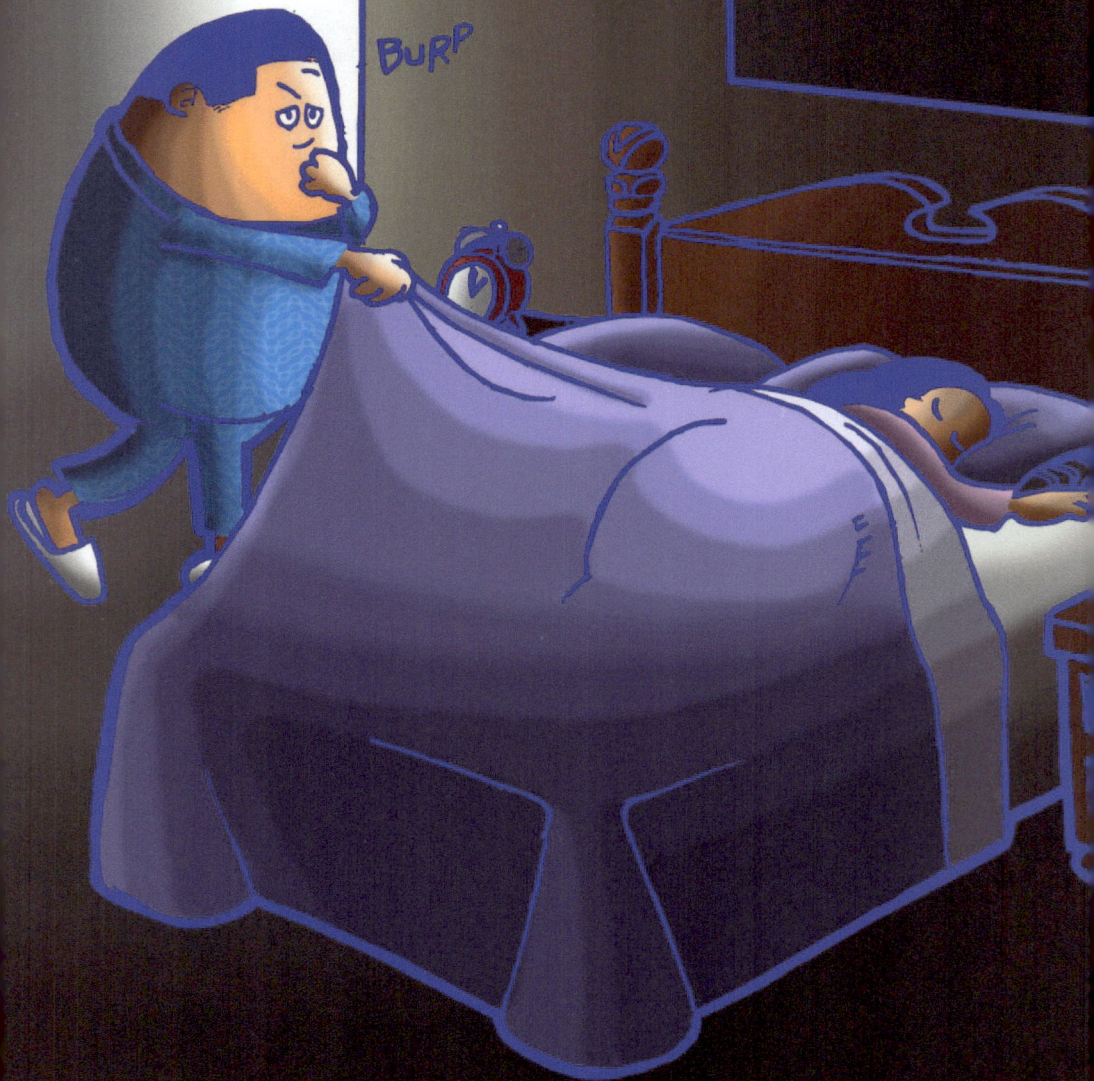

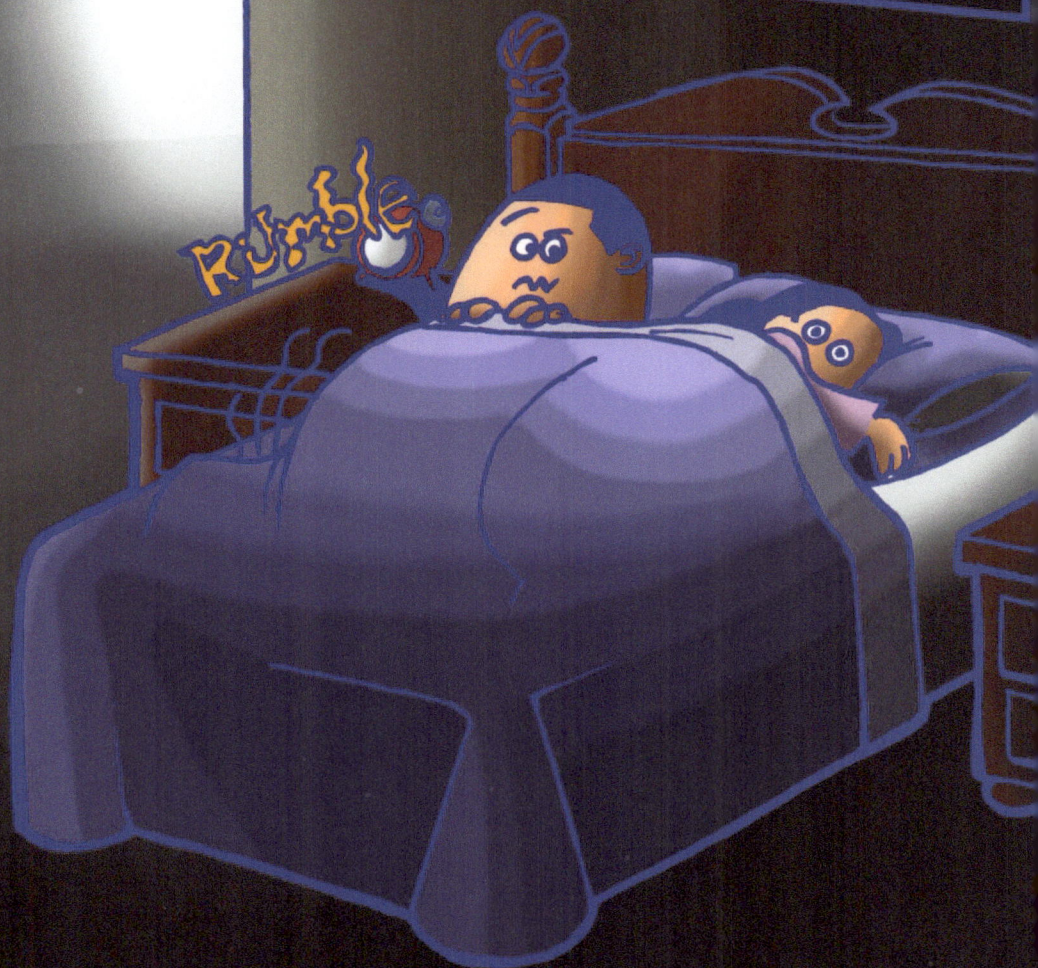

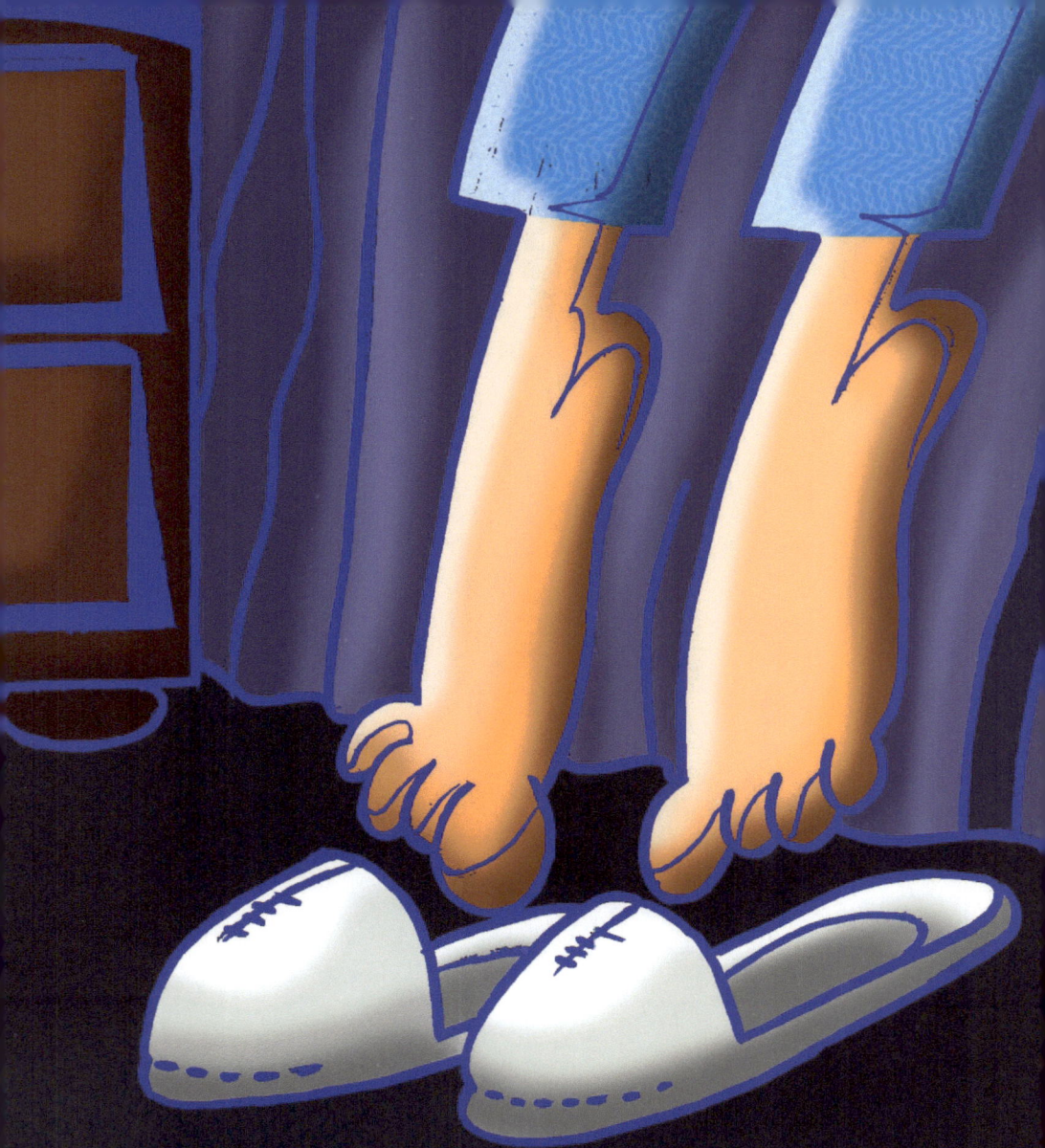

This time will be different.
Let's give it a try!

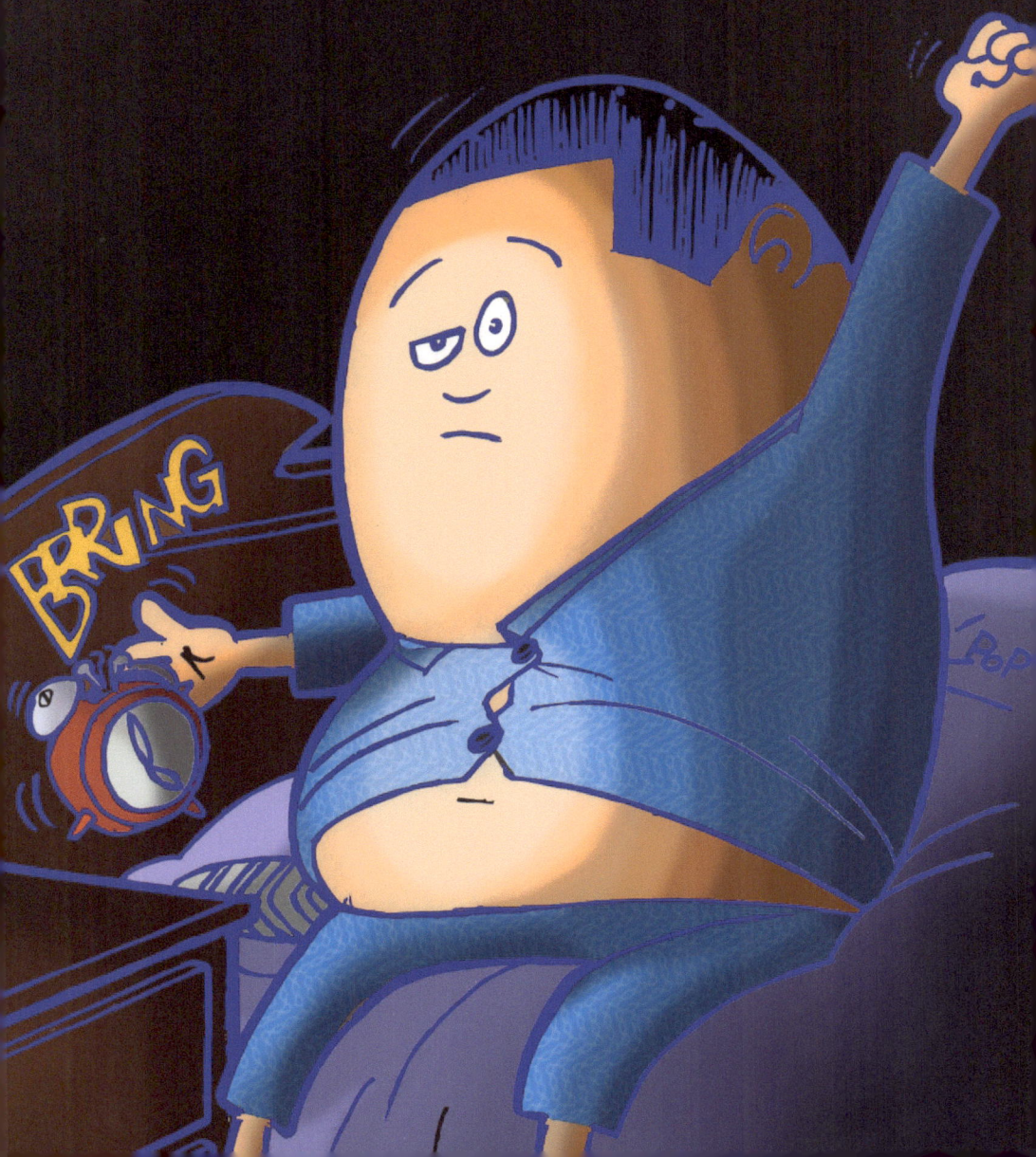

We need to get healthy.
I'll tell you why...

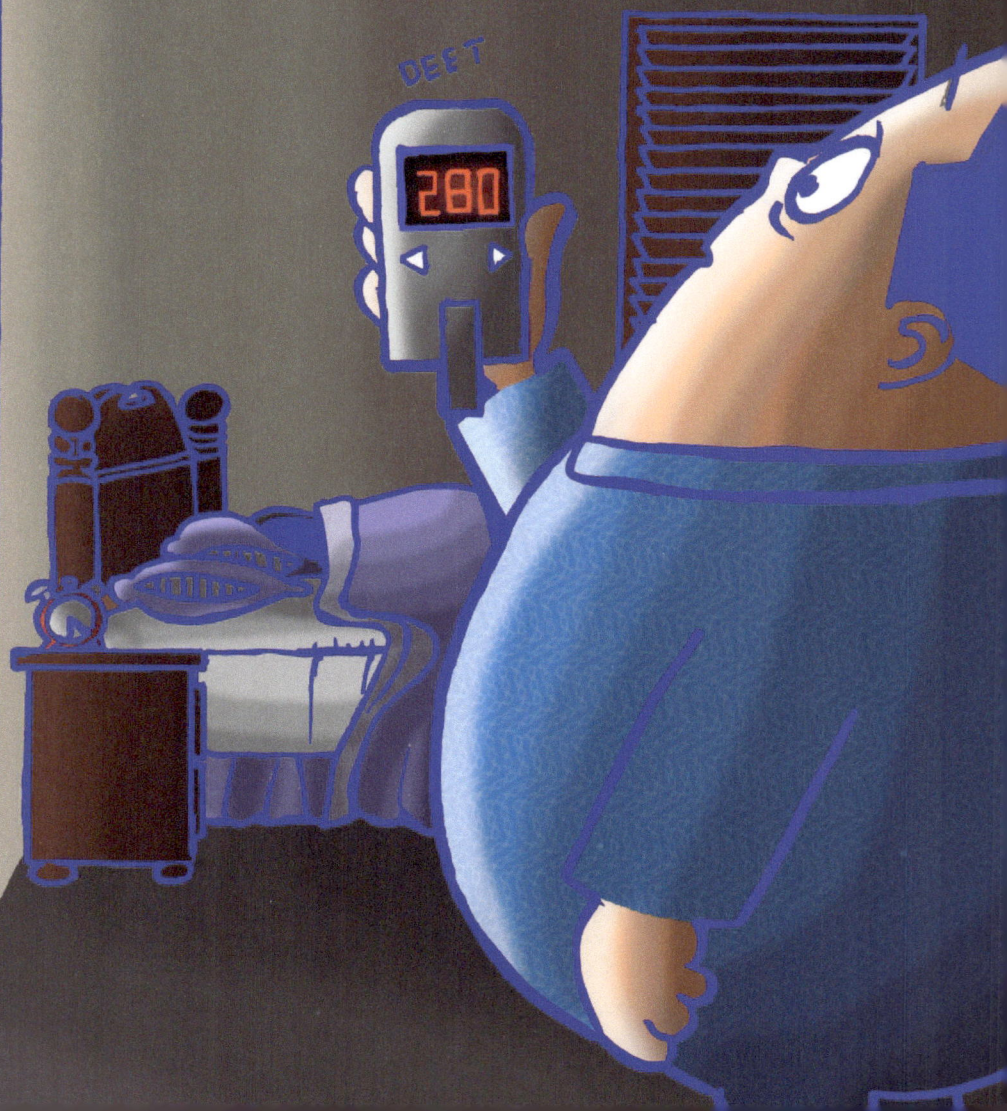

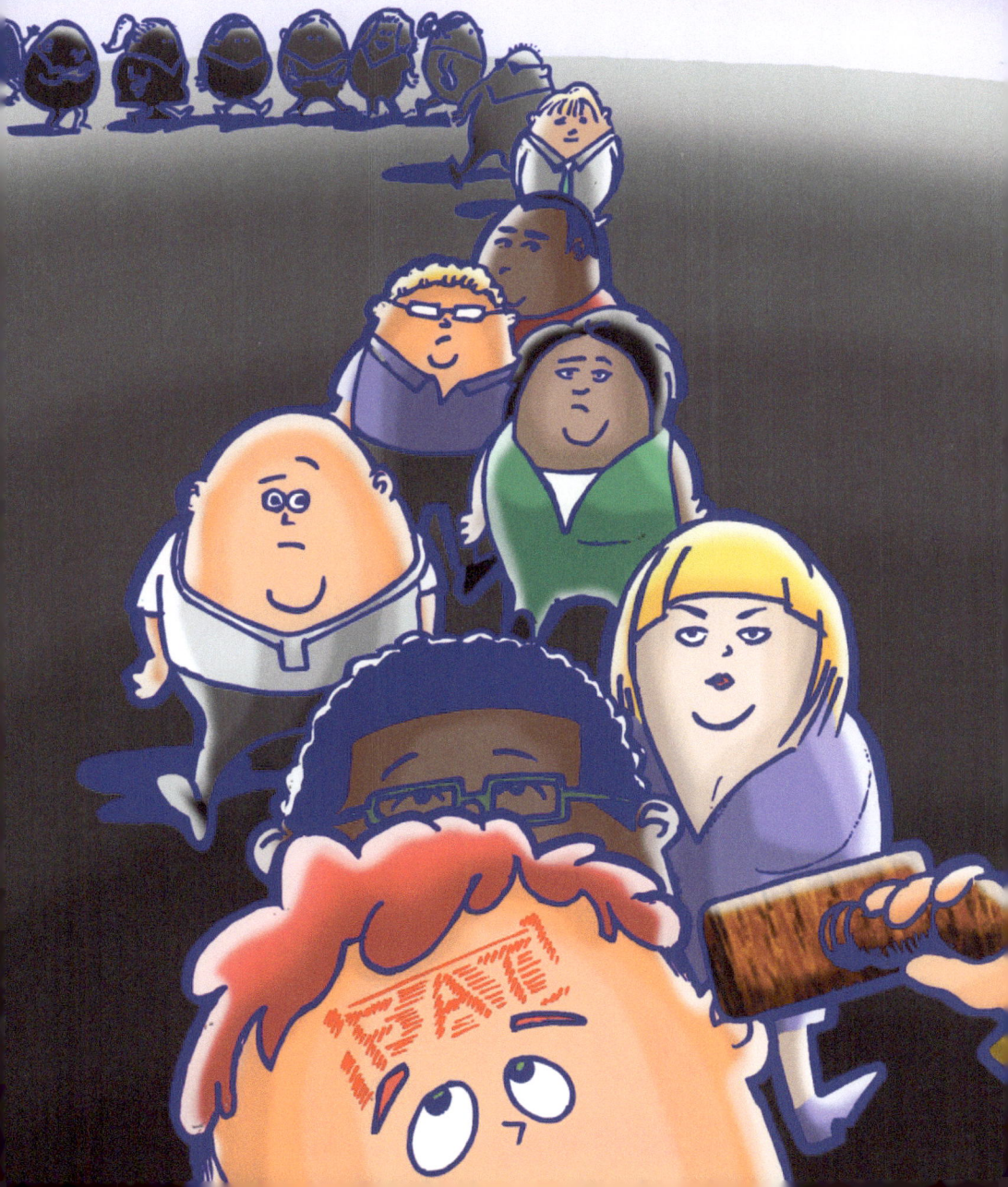

It's time to fight back!
Gotta take some control!

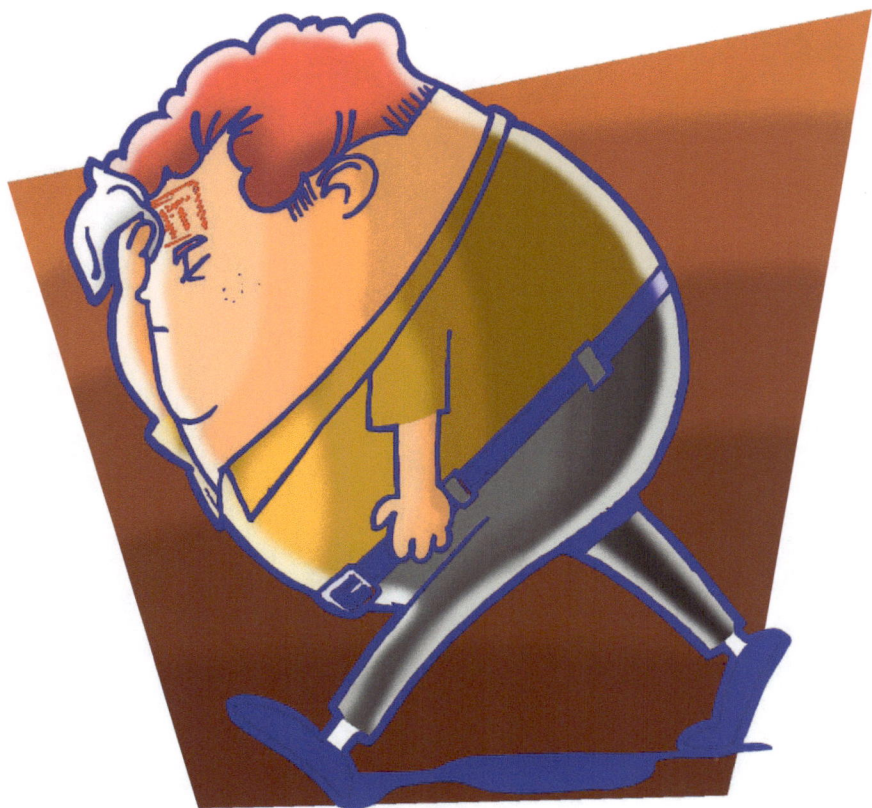

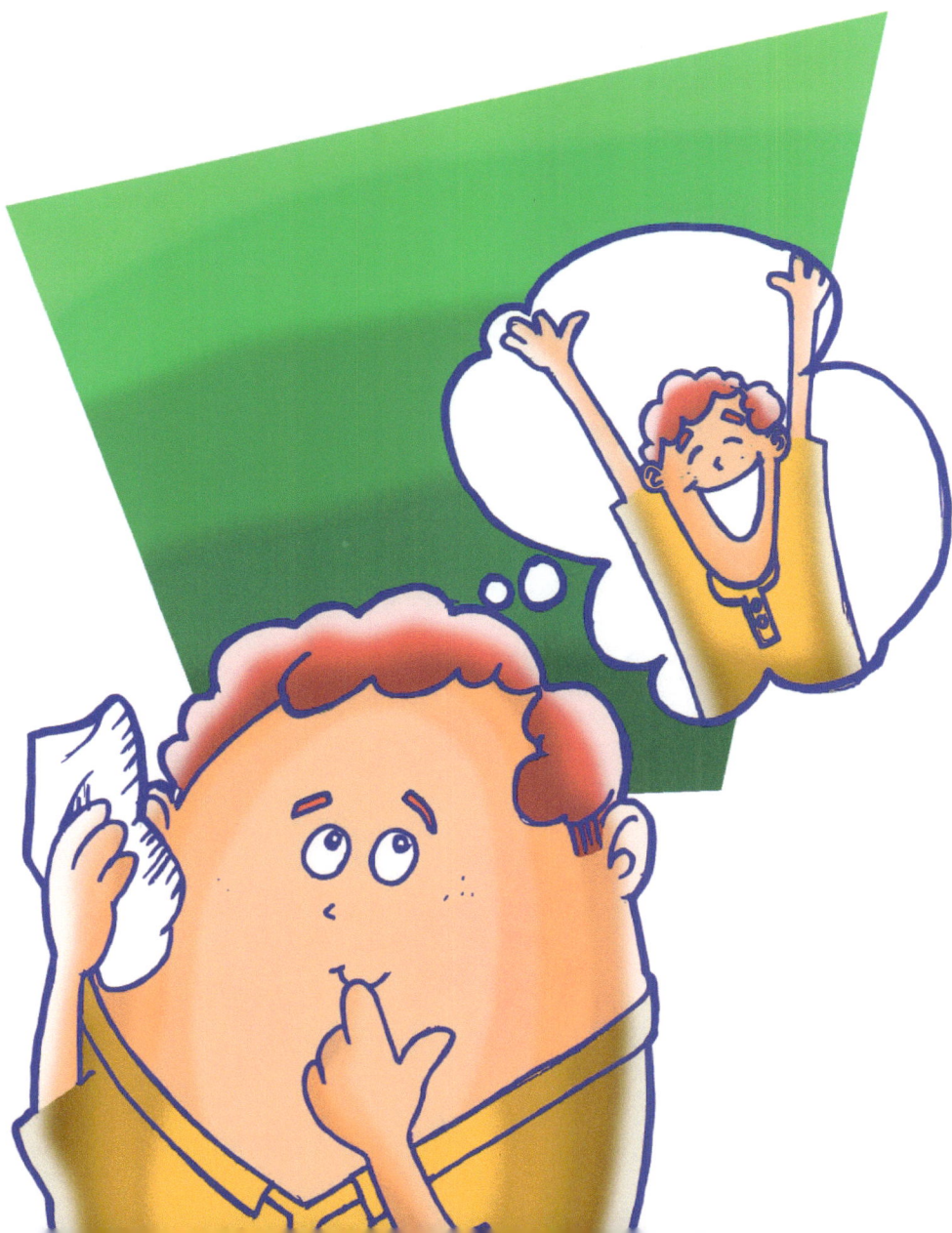

Let's throw out our candy, chips, cookies and cake.

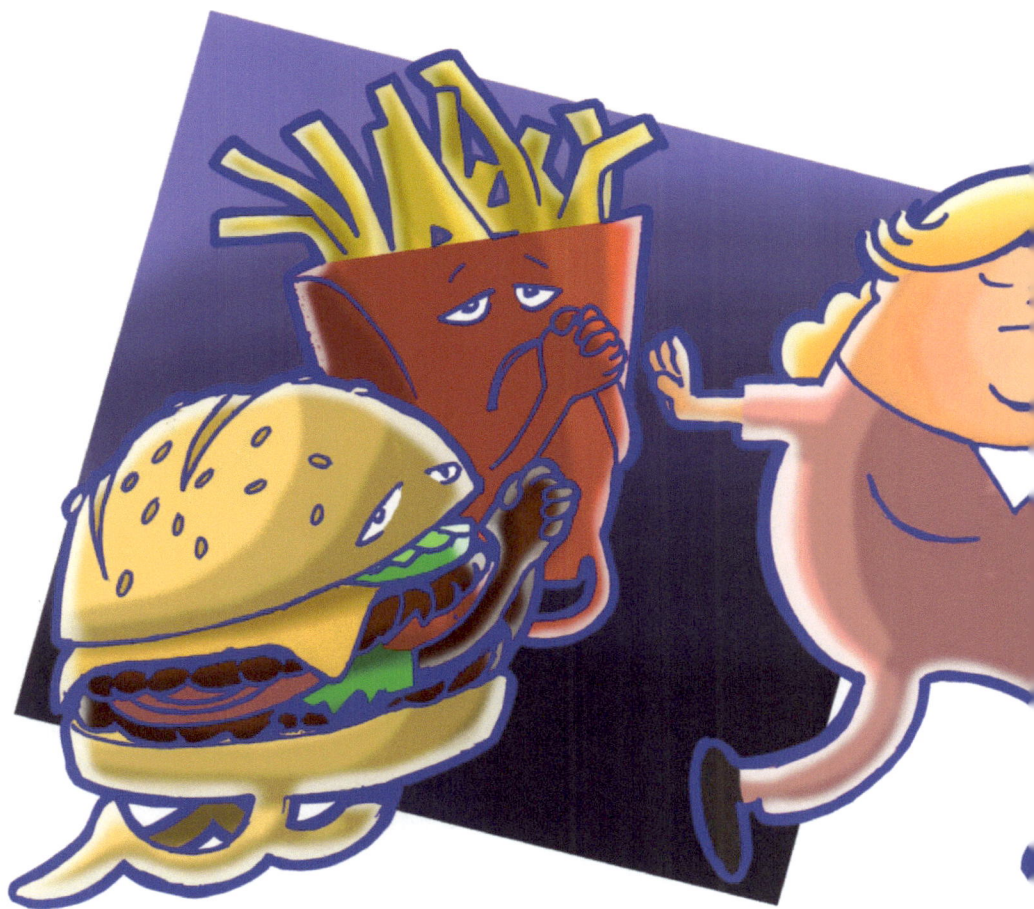

No more big burgers,
large fries or cheesesteak!

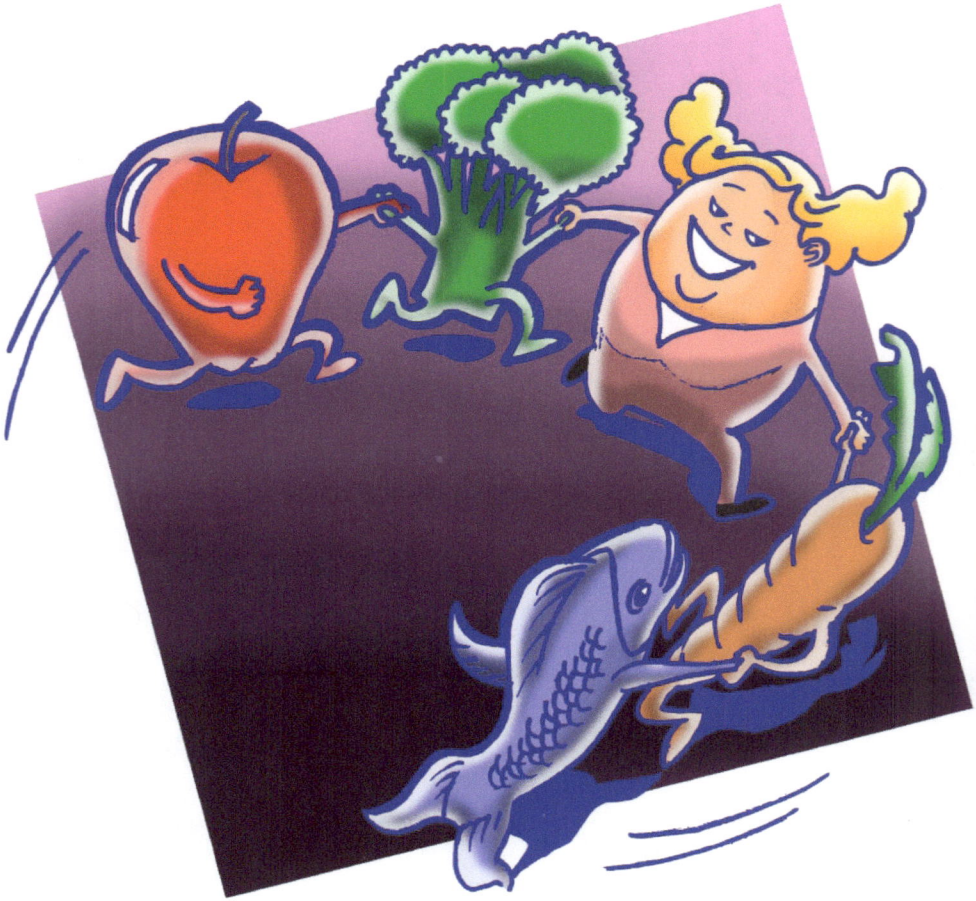

Replace them with
fruit, veggies, pasta and fish.

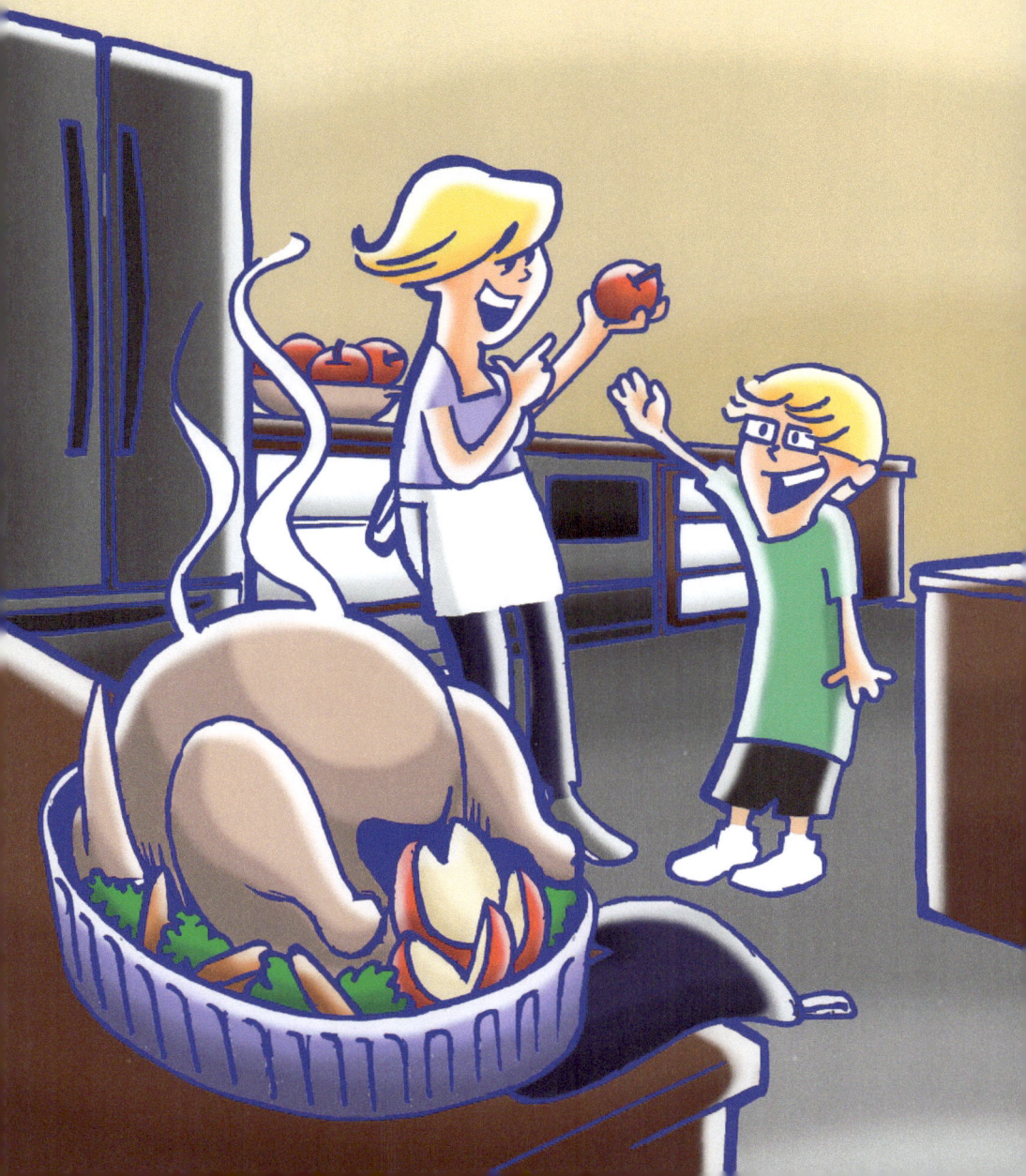

Whole grains and chicken,
we can eat what we wish!

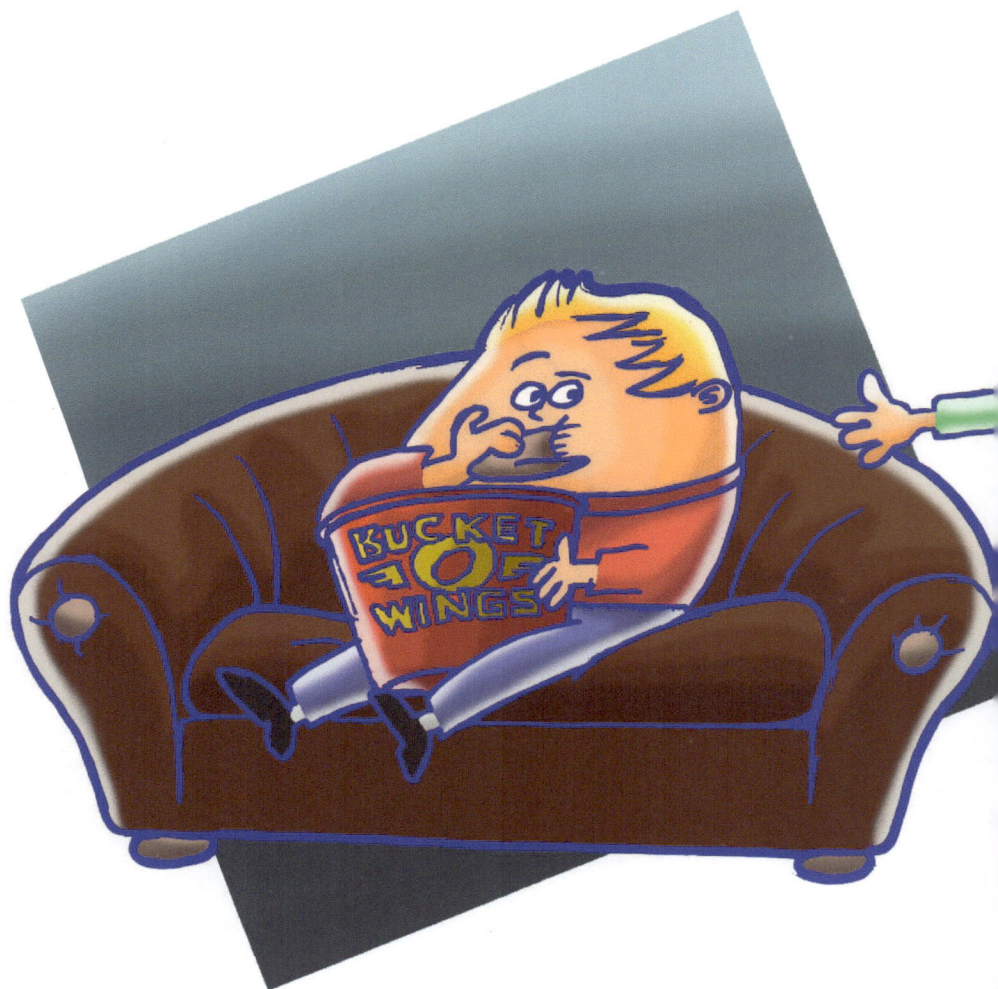

Let's get off the sofa
and get our hearts pumping!

Let's go for a jog,
then do some rope jumping!

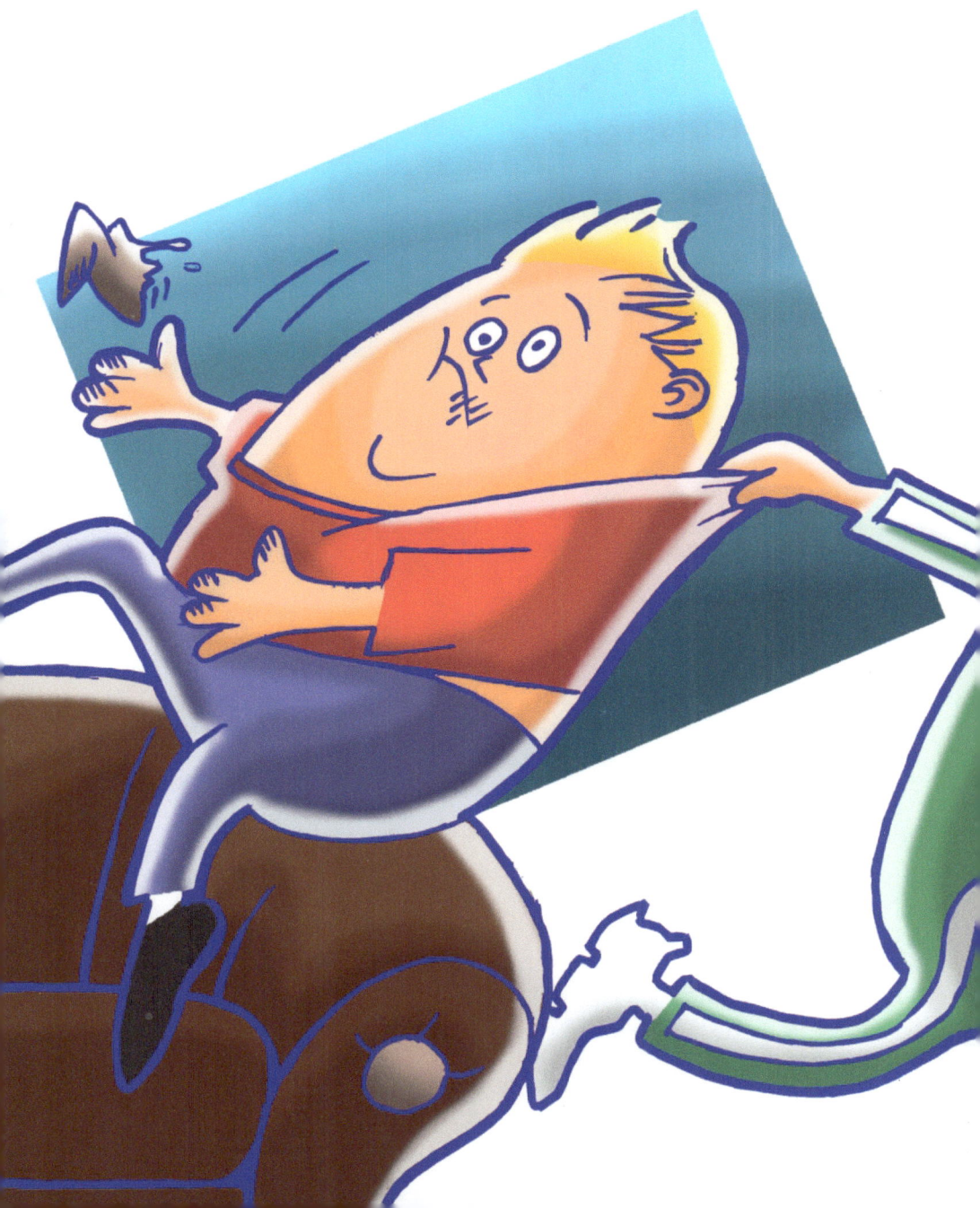

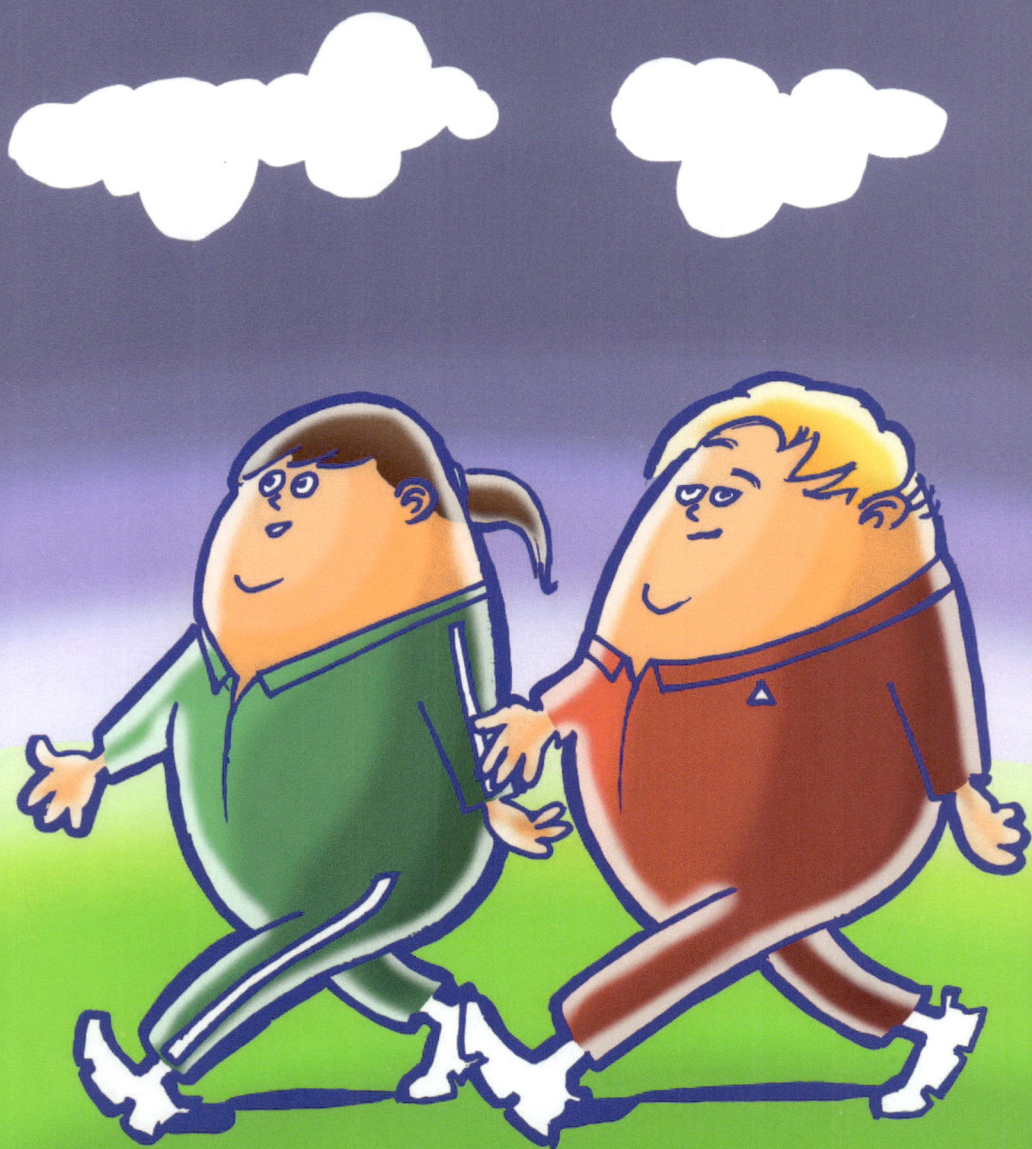

Let's go for a walk...

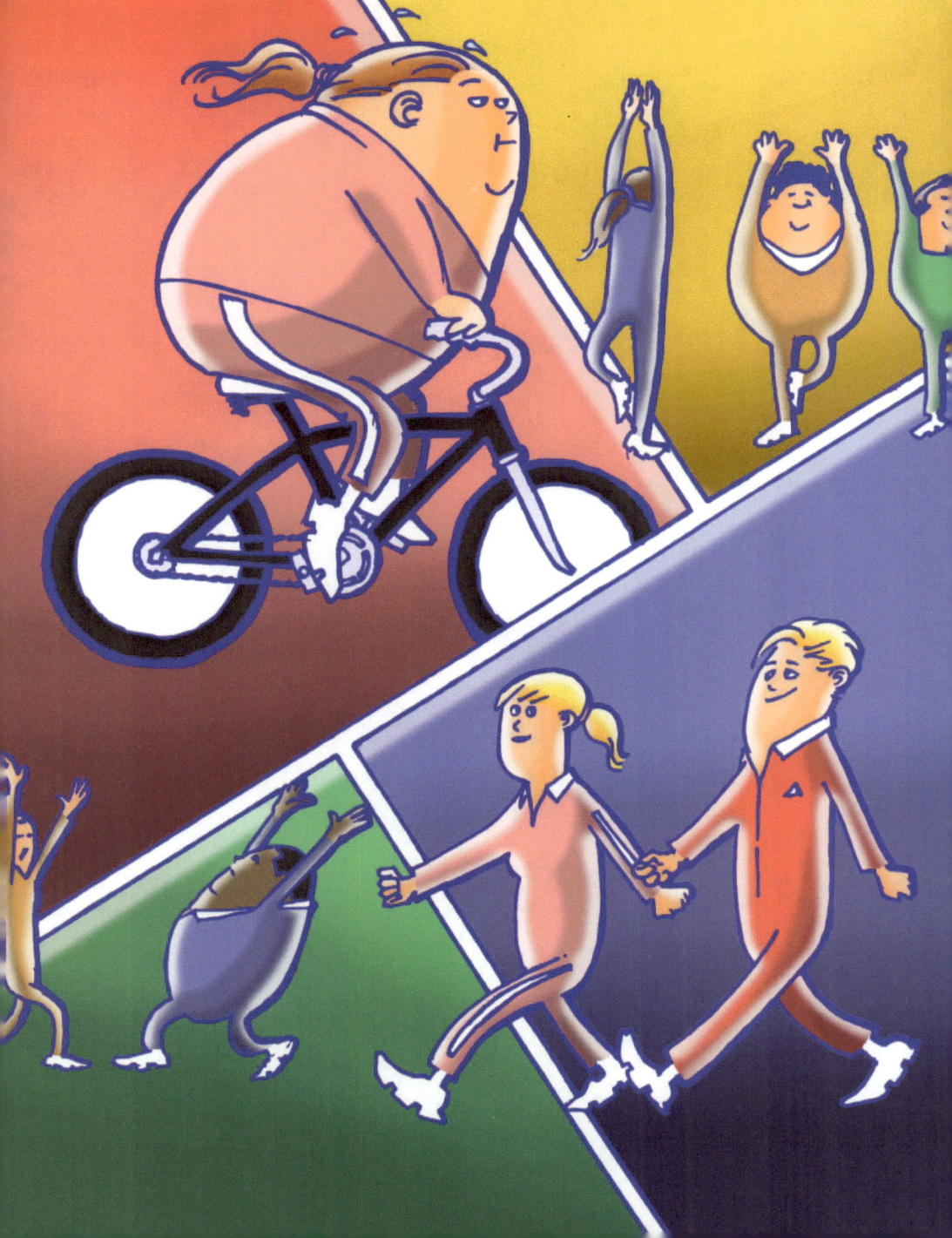

or take a
class at the gym.

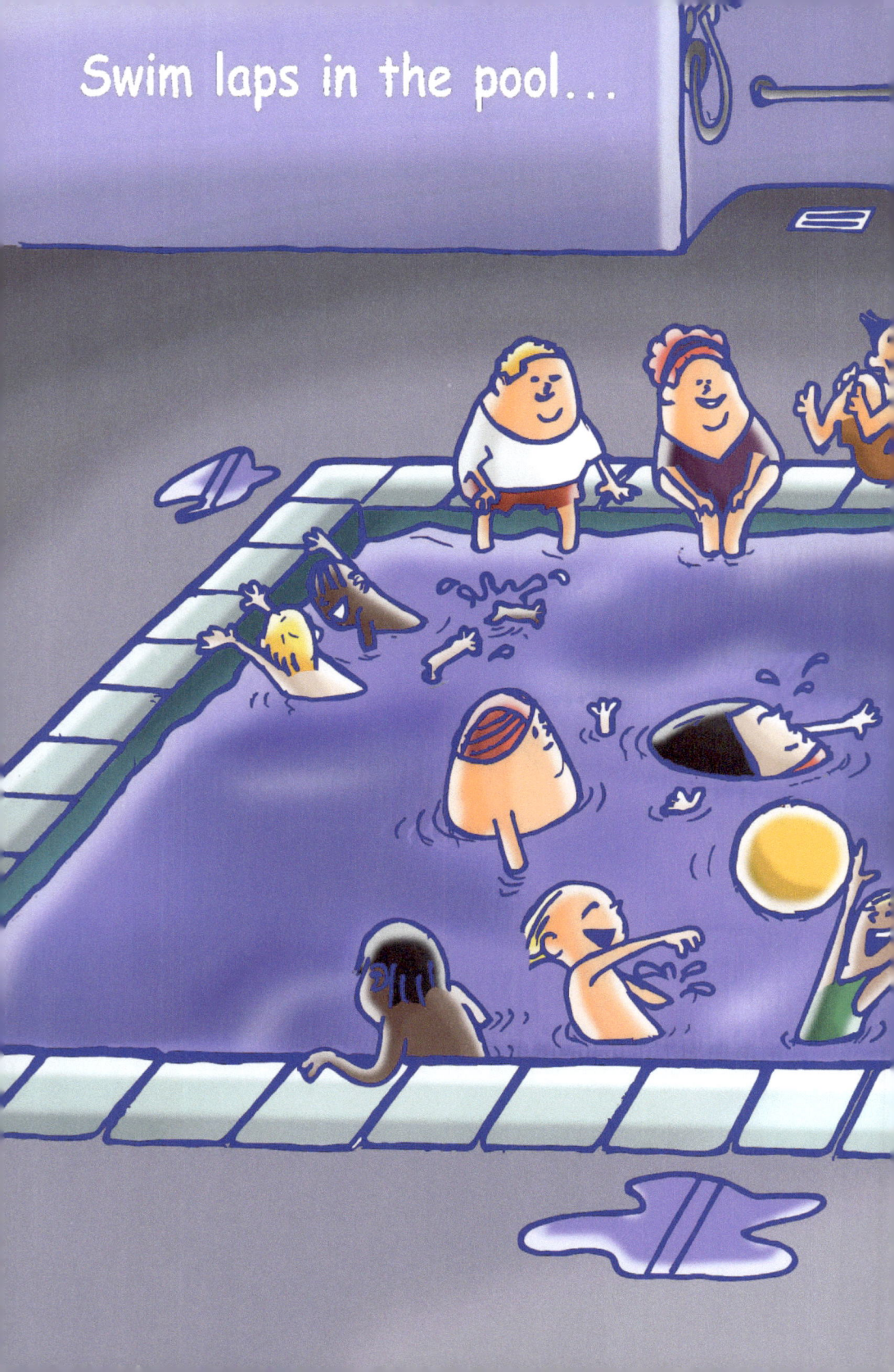

Swim laps in the pool...

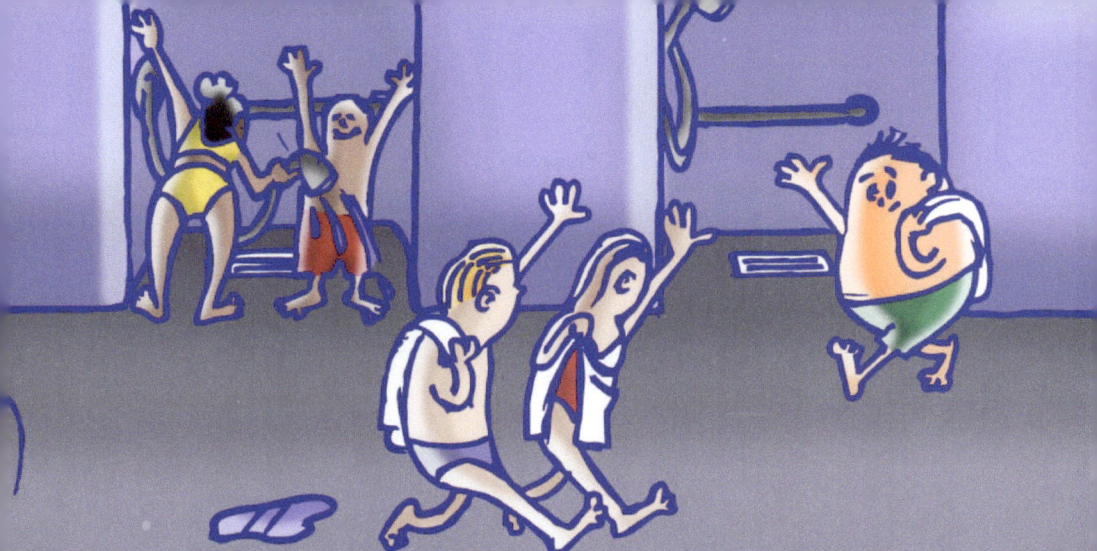

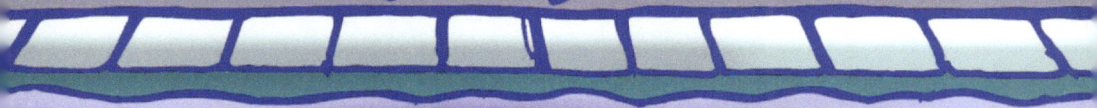

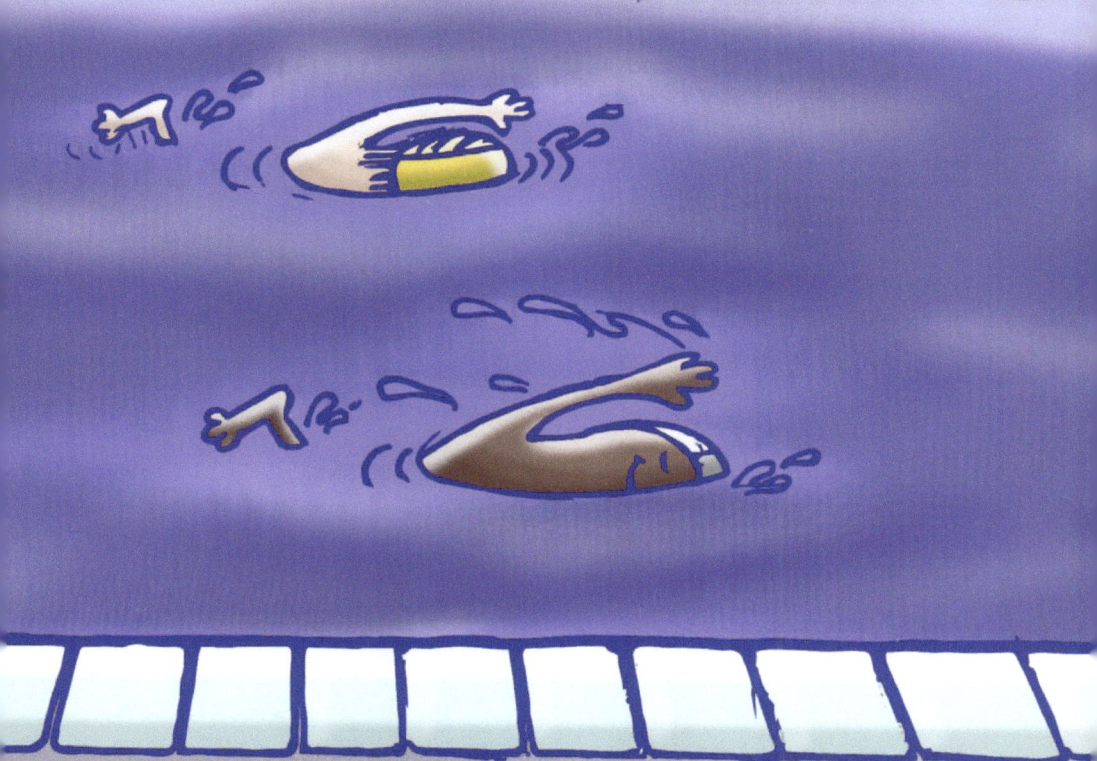

Let's start to get slim!

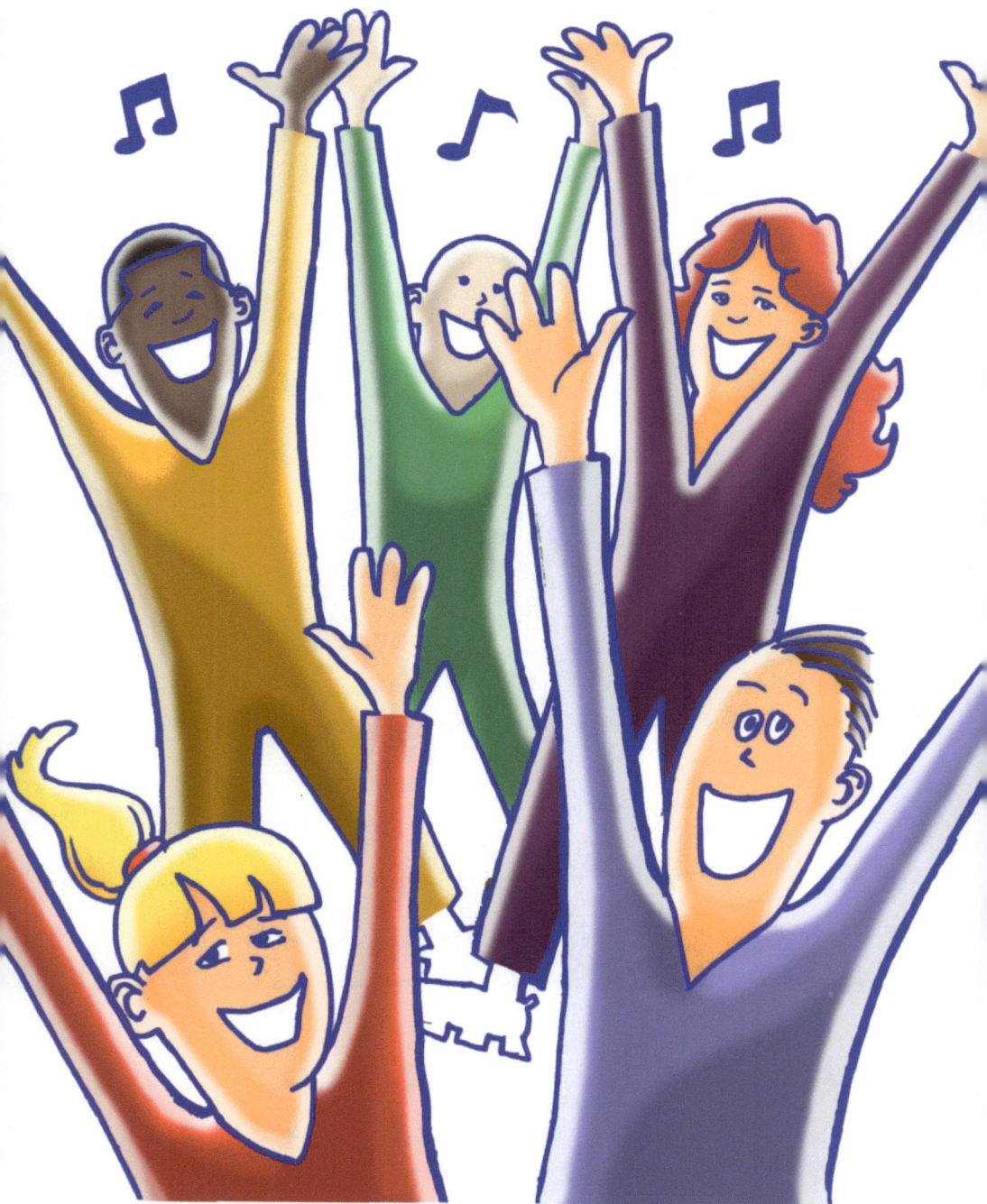

Get up and wake up!
Shake, dance or groove!

Quit being lazy! We just need to move

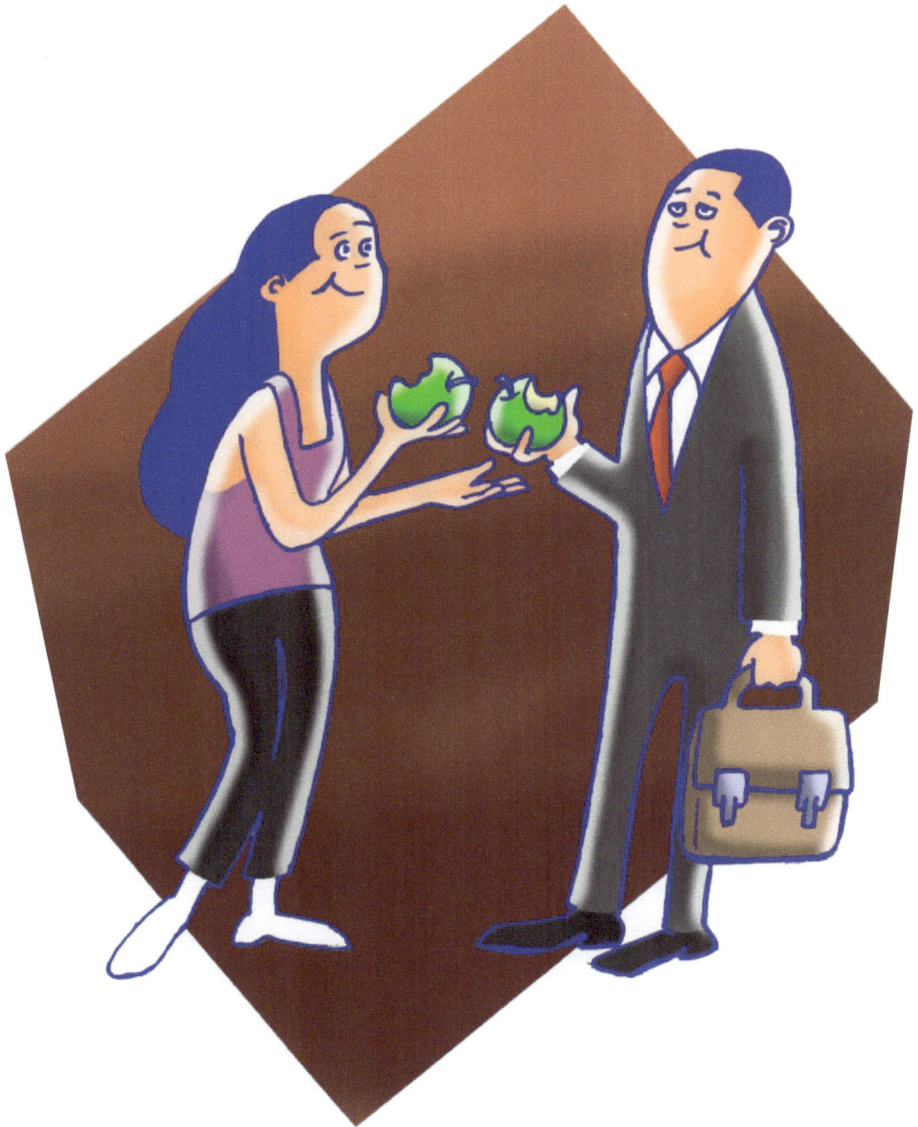

As soon as we do this,
we'll start to lose weight

We'll feel so much better.
We'll really look great!

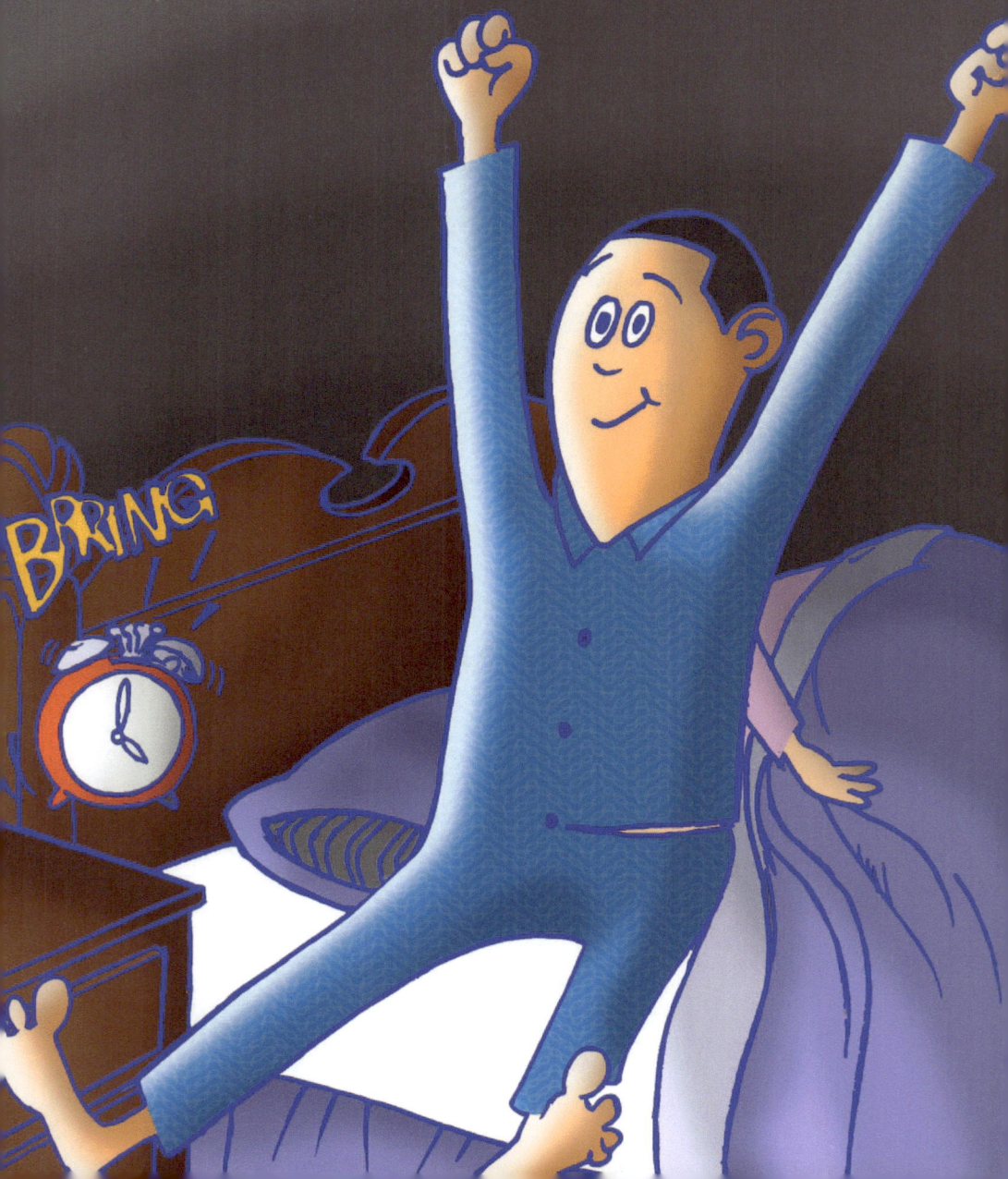

It's time to get healthy!
I know we can!

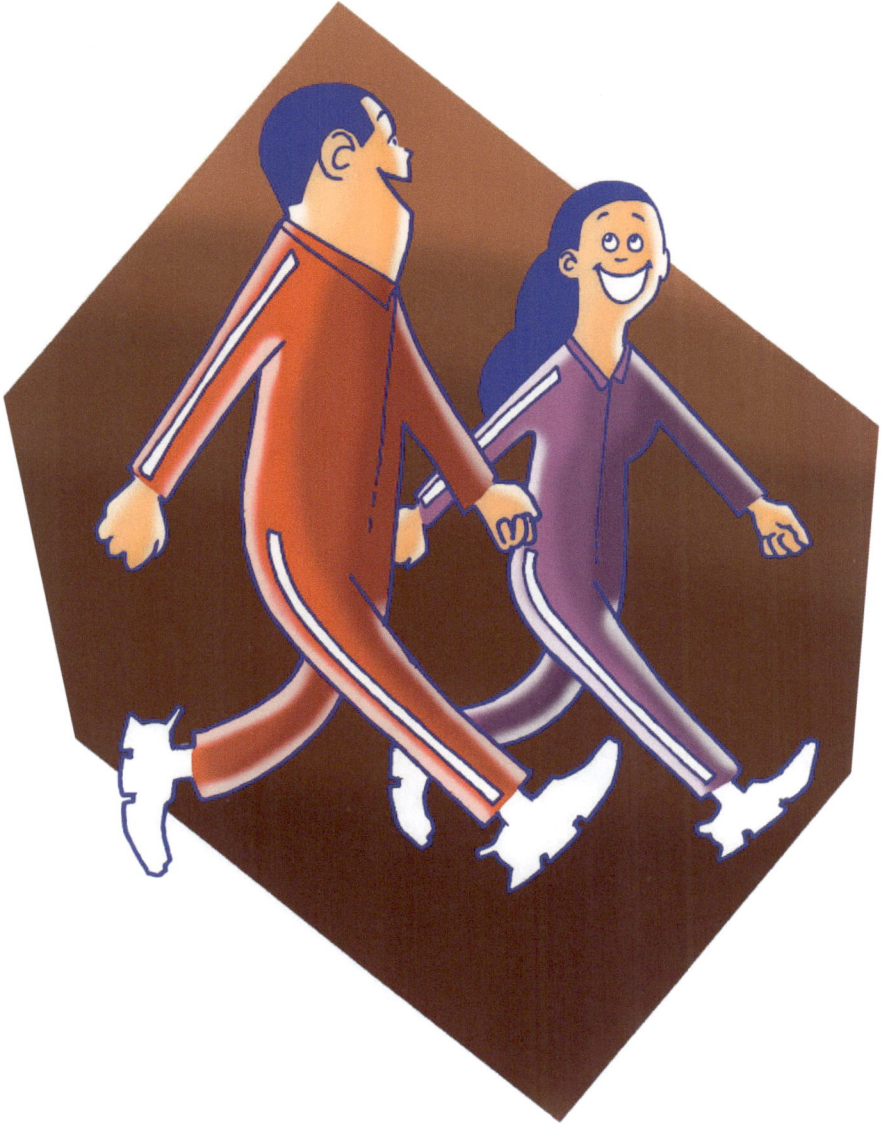

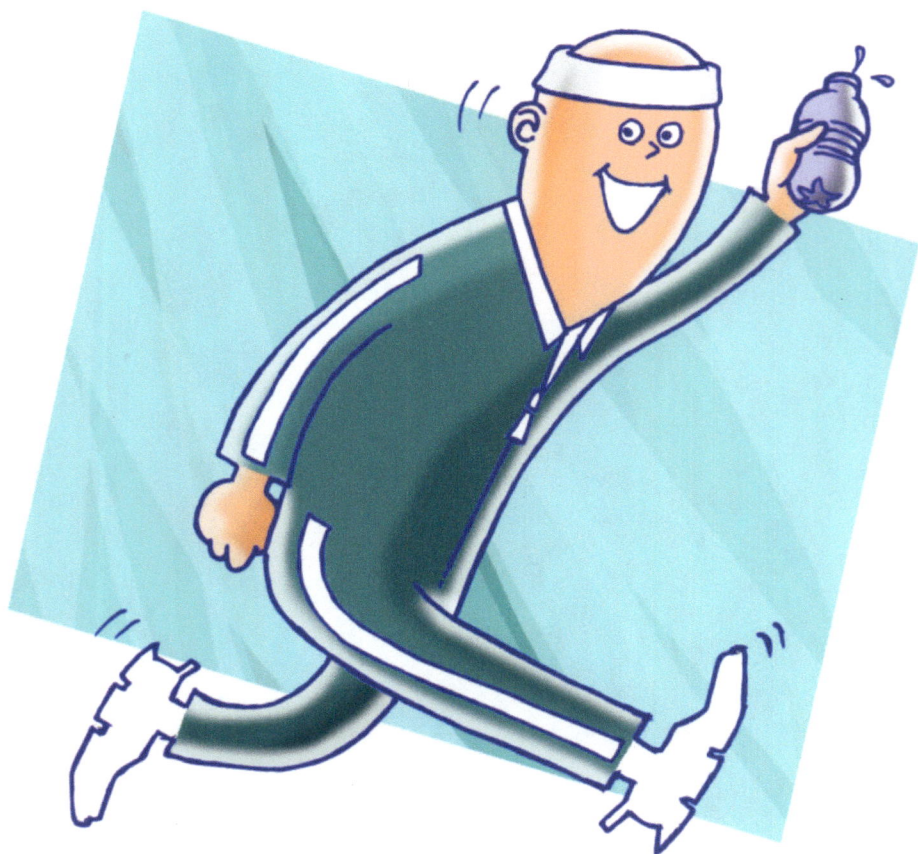

Come on America!
Let's take a stance!

We need to get healthy!
This is our chance!

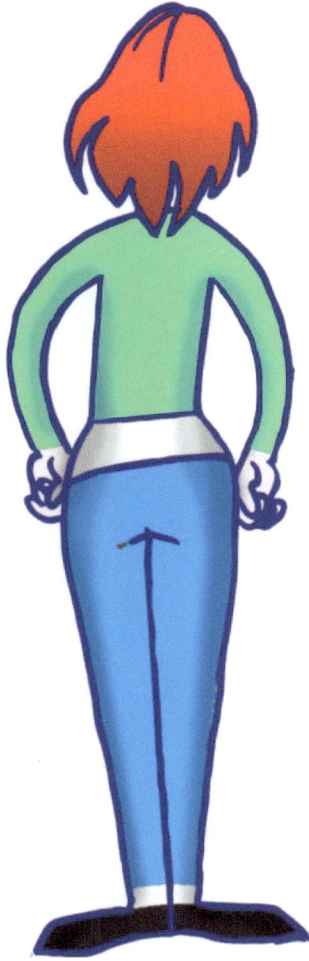

The End

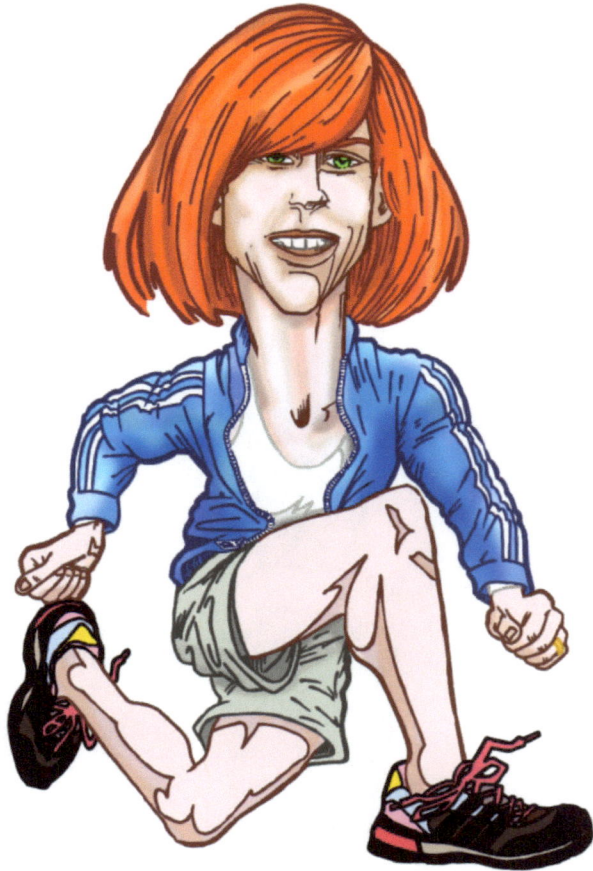

Kimberly Sandefur lives in Macon, GA with her husband, Terrell and twins, Nina and Wyatt. She has two dogs and a cat. Her hobbies include working-out and cooking. Most of the ideas for this book came to her while she was on her treadmill or power-walking in her neighborhood. She humorously refers to herself as The Red Rhymer.

www.ingramcontent.com/pod-product-compliance
Lightning Source LLC
Chambersburg PA
CBHW041222270326
41933CB00001B/16

9 780615 926513